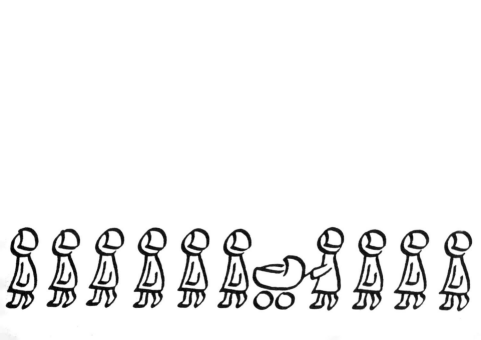

The One Girl in Ten

A Self Portrait of the Teen-age Mother

v

Sallie Foster

Child Welfare League of America, Inc.
440 First Street, NW, Suite 310, Washington, DC 20001-2085
(202)638-2952

Current Printing (last digit)
10 9 8 7 6 5 4 3 2
Printed in the United States of America

ISBN # 0-87868-343-7

Title Page and Cover Design by Ann Doskow

Acknowledgments

I want to thank a number of people for the help and encouragement they have given me in the preparation of this book:

The Board of Directors of Gateway House in Pomona, California, for their continued interest in the project since its earliest beginnings.

The Claremont Foundation, for the grant which made it possible to carry out the project.

Teachers of special programs for pregnant girls in various school districts of Los Angeles and San Bernardino counties, and other professionals, who provided me an introduction to young mothers they knew: Miriam Ades, Merle Church, Barbara Evans, Laura Hoffman, Mary Lewis, Jeanne Lindsay, Jeen Nelson, Estella Patch, Ethel Ripley, Dorothy Walker, Millie Weiss, Myrna Wheeler, Mary Lou Williams, Polly Wilson, and Alice Youngquist.

Beverly Wachel and Nancy Sasse, who spent hundreds of hours transcribing the taped interviews.

Shirley Kemper and Ruth Hail, who provided expert secretarial assistance in the preparation of the manuscript.

Members of my family, and the following friends and former colleagues who read the manuscript, in whole or in part, and made helpful suggestions: Annette Crowell, Margaret Faust, Beth Hadady, Lynn Piatt, Corinne Smith, Bill Stelzner, and Marion Stewart.

Finally, I want to express my thanks to every one of those remarkable young mothers who adopted this project as their very own, and admitted me to their hearts as well as their homes. No words can adequately express my feelings for them, or my indebtedness to them. All I can say is—this is *their* book.

Sallie Foster

Contents

CHAPTER ONE

The Story behind the Statistics

This is not a book about teen-age pregnancy as a "national problem" or a "social phenomenon." It is a book about *people* — people who have had the experience of becoming pregnant, and bearing children, while they were very young. It is a story, rather than a study — *their* story. It will present no charts or graphs or tables, but instead will simply let the reader know what happened, what various people thought, what they did, and especially how they felt, as events were taking place which were to change the course of their lives and the lives of those around them.

Quite often, when a young girl becomes pregnant, her family surrounds her with a cloak of secrecy while they try to resolve the complex problems such a situation always creates. It is painful for them to talk about it, and so they are apt to confide only in a few close friends or relatives. Consequently, most people have very little understanding of teen-age pregnancy, except in general terms — until it occurs in their own family.

One mistaken notion which has been widely accepted is the assumption that when teen-agers become pregnant they all rush to get abortions. The facts, however, do not bear this out. Although about one third choose to have abortions, the majority choose to continue their pregnancies, and most of them keep their babies.

In this book attention is focused on the experiences of girls who were eighteen or younger when they had their babies — the "school age mothers." By virtue of numbers alone, they form an important segment of society, for every year nearly a quarter of a million additional young mothers join this group. It is estimated that *one girl in ten will give birth to a child before she reaches her eighteenth birthday.*

After working with hundreds of school age mothers as a social worker, I had become familiar with the crisis which an unexpected pregnancy precipitates. Invariably, when I made the first home call and began talking with family members, I found them in a state of shock. No one—not even the girl herself—had expected this to happen. They seemed unable to think clearly or make any plans. Feelings were all that mattered, and they were so intense and so palpable that they completely overshadowed any conversation that took place.

As the years went by, it occurred to me that people would have a clearer understanding of teen-age pregnancy if they could just listen, as I had listened so often, to those who had been through this experience themselves. I decided to see if some young mothers would be willing to tell their stories, and let others have the benefit of their first-hand accounts.

Finding girls who were willing to be interviewed proved to be an easier task than might have been expected. Through the teachers of special classes for pregnant girls offered in various school districts under a special state program in California, I found many young mothers who wanted very much to participate in this project, and over a twelve-month period I recorded 126 interviews on tape.

In order to talk with the girls in a setting that was familiar to them, I usually went to their homes, which were located in small towns and cities scattered over a broad area lying to the east of the City of Los Angeles.

Though no specific questions were asked regarding family income or ethnic origin, a brief description of the group that participated, in general terms, may be of interest to the reader. Most of the girls came from "middle class" families living in residential neighborhoods. More than half the group were white, over twenty-five per cent were Mexican-American, and about ten per cent were black, reflecting rather closely the incidence of these major ethnic groups in the communities visited.

At the time of the interviews, the girls were between fifteen and twenty-four years of age, and the ages of their first-born children ranged from six weeks to six years. The girls had only one characteristic in common: *they had all had a child while they were still of school age.* Twenty-five of them had been fifteen or younger when they first gave birth.

The girls were friendly, and they were refreshingly frank. It sometimes seemed as if they had been waiting a long time for a chance to tell their stories, and had been keeping their real feelings bottled up tight. They had a great many things on their minds, and they did not hesitate to say them. They wanted to tell other girls what they had gone through. They also wanted to tell other girls' parents some things they had never been able to tell their own parents.

Out of more than five thousand pages of tape transcripts came the material for this book. The feelings of the girls, their relationship to parents and boy friends, their attitudes toward the various alternative decisions open to them, and their opinions about important people in their lives, like doctors, clergymen, teachers, and social workers—all are presented in considerable detail in an attempt to increase general understanding of the conditions which cause a very young girl to become a mother. In describing their own experiences the girls have produced a composite picture of the school age mother—the teen-ager who, once she has become pregnant, chooses to bear her child and keep it.

This book is not a complete or objective discussion of all the factors which are involved in early parenthood. It presents the *girls'* point of view. Since they were the only ones interviewed, all other persons mentioned in the book are described as seen through their eyes. Similarly, the chapters on abortion, adoption, marriage, the school, and the church do not purport to be objective discussions of these subjects; rather, they present the attitudes of particular girls toward these matters at a specific time in their lives when they suddenly assumed special importance.

Although many important topics were discussed during the course of the interviews, the scope of this book necessitated restricting the selection of material to certain subjects associated with a particular time in each girl's life—from the time of her first sexual experience, through the crisis produced by the pregnancy, to the period after childbirth.

Names have been changed to protect the privacy of the girls who were interviewed. If any story in this book sounds familiar to a particular reader, however, I will not be surprised, for though the young women who speak were all living in Southern California, their counterparts can be found in every neighborhood, in every town, in every state in this country.

CHAPTER TWO

The Shock of Discovery

We usually started our conversations with this question: Could they remember how they felt when they first discovered they were pregnant? Whether this question took them back in time only a couple of months, or several years, it always evoked an emotional response. They did remember. One girl said quite simply, "I remember everything."

Were they happy when they realized they were pregnant? Some were—usually those who were planning to marry the father of the baby. There were others whose reasons for being happy were less obvious, but none the less genuine; for example, one girl who was tired of running said, "I wanted something to tie me down. I wanted something that depended on me. I wanted that."

Others said they were happy—but only *partly*. "I had been wanting to get pregnant," one of the girls said quite frankly. Then she thought a moment, and amended her statement in a curious way: "But not really—I wanted to get pregnant, but I didn't want to have a baby." And then, as if she were turning this idea over in her mind, she repeated the statement: "I wanted to get pregnant—but I didn't want to have a baby."

For the overwhelming majority, however, the realization that they were indeed pregnant came as a profound shock.

I was really startled. I thought, "It couldn't happen to me." My life had gone smoothly up until that point. Everything went really nice. In junior high I was president of the student body. I helped teach catechism. Then in high school I was in drill team—always involved in things. And I just thought, "This can't happen to *me!* There's got to be some mistake."

Before they had any medical proof they were pregnant, many had been able to figure out the situation for themselves and were reasonably sure they *were;* yet this growing conviction, instead of spurring them to action, had the opposite effect. They could not believe what they suspected, and they did everything they could think of to avoid consulting anyone who could tell them for sure. They made up their own explanations for the way they felt, or consulted friends. Anything seemed preferable to going to a doctor.

Even morning sickness, which is frequently a symptom of early pregnancy, was sometimes given another interpretation.

Well, I'd heard about it, you know, morning sickness, and—I missed so much school! Like, I would be on my way to school and I'd get sick and everything. I kind of had a feeling that I was pregnant, but I wasn't sure, you know. It was just one of those things. I wasn't terribly worried—not really—because I thought, "Not me, it can't happen to me." So I figured it was probably just the flu.

Without doubt, the physical symptoms of pregnancy were at times extremely confusing.

My period was real irregular, I'd skip five months at a time. And then I had a bathing suit on one day, and—well, I was *thinner* than I was before! But I told my mom that I was getting scared because I hadn't had my period and she said, "Well, you're not pregnant, because I can tell by the way you look." And so we went to the free clinic first and they told me I wasn't pregnant. Then I went to my doctor and told her what they had said, so she ran all kinds of tests for diabetes and she gave me a complete physical, and she said, "Marilyn, you're more than five months pregnant."

Even a mature woman would find the following circumstances bewildering, but they were especially difficult for a fifteen-year-old girl to comprehend.

I had my period until my seventh month of pregnancy, and so that made it very difficult for us to know. I had morning sickness and I figured, "Well, I must be pregnant," but then when my period came, I thought, "Oh, I'm not." And I started swelling, but then I was losing weight, so then I figured, "Well, I can't be."

I was sick. I played volleyball and softball, and I lost a lot of weight, and I was just so sick. Just miserably sick.

My mom used to ask me if I thought I was pregnant, and I told her, "No, I couldn't be." And so finally one day she picked me up from school, and she decided we'd better go down to the doctor's and check, because I was so sick. And so we went down and sure enough, I was six months.

Once in a while a doctor actually added to the general confusion, as in the following case. The girl was certain she was pregnant, and her mother suspected she was, too, but could not bear the thought of it.

She didn't want to take me to the family doctor, because she didn't want to be embarrassed. She heard about this other doctor from a friend at work—he was a quack, believe me. She said, "I'm going to take you to the doctor, because for you being so sick, if you're not pregnant, then something else is wrong with you."

So then I went, and the dumb doctor that she took me to thought I had gallstones. 'Cause he was pressing my stomach, he felt a lump, but he didn't think that it was a baby. So then he told me that he wanted to see how many gallstones I had, and how big they were.

I wanted to laugh, because I knew that I didn't have gallstones, you know. And I said to myself, "Well, if they think that I have gallstones, I just won't take the medicine they give me and I still won't tell them." But then he wanted to give me some kind of solution, this dye, to drink to color the gallstones so when they put me in an x-ray it would fill them in and they could see dark spots. And I thought, "No, what happens if that hurts the baby?" And I told my mom, "I don't have gallstones," and she goes, "Well, if the doctor says you do, you do. What else is wrong with you?" And I told her. Then she said, "I don't believe you." The doctor said, "Are you sure?" And I said, "Yeah." My mom goes, "I don't think she knows what's wrong with her."

And so he gave me a blood test and a urine test to see if I was pregnant, and said he would call the next day.

People who are determined to avoid finding out the truth are apt to grab onto any explanation that offers even a temporary reprieve. Just as Yvonne did.

All my life my weight has gone up and down, up and down. So I just said, "Well, maybe I'm gaining weight," because I didn't want to admit it to myself that I was pregnant. So I just said, "No, I'm gaining weight, I'm gaining weight." So I went to the free clinic, to get a pregnancy test. But at the time I had been going to those doctors, you know, those fast-reducing doctors, who give you a shot—that HCG—anyways, it's the same thing as the pregnant woman's urine. That's what it is. And so when I told them that I was going to that doctor, they said, "Oh, it could give you a false reading." They told me to come back, and they'd give me a different test.

And I didn't want to go back. I didn't want to know that I was. So I just kept telling myself, "I'm not. I'm not. I'm not." Until I felt the kicking, and I said, "Oh, brother!" And I just—I don't know. I still didn't do anything about it. I didn't tell my mom I was pregnant until my ninth month. And I never went to the doctor's.

The steadfast denial of something that is becoming a more and more obvious reality requires constant vigilance and considerable ingenuity. The types of action taken to conceal a pregnancy resemble what is commonly called a "cover-up," because they stem from the same strong motivating force—*fear*. Sometimes the fear is specific: "What will my parents say?" "Will my boy friend leave me?" Often it includes a general fear of the unknown. But always it is powerful, capable of stifling all appropriate action and producing symptoms of serious depression.

It is by no means normal for a fifteen-year-old girl to withdraw from her family for as long as Molly did, yet in all that time no one tried to find out why.

My boy friend went off and I didn't have nobody to talk to so I just sat around at home. And I didn't want my dad to find out, so I just stayed in my room. For about six months I stayed in my room the whole time.

I would forget to eat a lot. Like I would just go to school and I would come home and I wouldn't eat, and I'd clean the house real fast, and then I'd go to my room and just pretend I was asleep, and I'd forget to eat. Or I'd just sit around drinking iced tea all day. And that's why I lost so much weight and everything.

The loneliness which Molly felt was described in more detail by another girl, who had vivid memories of a very hard time in her life, and how she survived it.

When I was pregnant, I'd lay in bed at night, and it was like being locked away in a very cold dungeon — no way to get out. You feel like yelling out, "Hey! Doesn't anybody care?" And I laid in there, and I realized that nobody really did care — at the time I really thought that nobody did care. You always wonder to yourself, "How do you stop the hurt, how do you stop the pain, how do you stop crying when you want to so bad, how do you stop being so hard, how do you stop being sour against people and everything else?" And it's hard, it really is. You wonder what you're going to do, how you're going to make it from day to day ... I used to live on dreams — they used to help me get through these things — but I'm not a dreamer any more. I've grown up, and I must say it's the hardest thing I've ever done — is growing up. When you get pregnant, you have to grow up fast.

More often than perhaps is generally realized, the virtual paralysis caused by denial, depression, and loneliness continues until time runs out. This is most apt to happen in the case of very young girls. The illustration which follows represents just such a situation. At the time of our conversation more than four years had passed since the birth of the child, but the memory of this experience, which had occurred when Ellie was only twelve years old, was very much alive.

I didn't have nobody to turn to, you know—like, I was afraid of my dad, and I couldn't tell my mom because, I don't know, I couldn't tell her. I don't know. So, I was going to have an abortion, and I had it all set up, and I went down there and I just couldn't do it, I just couldn't do it. I just kept putting it off, and putting it off. And then finally it became too late and the first time that I went to see a doctor about the abortion he told me that it was too late, and that I couldn't have it. And he asked me, I remember him asking me, "Do you want me to take care of you, be your doctor, give you prenatal care?" I was dumb, and I didn't even know what that meant, and I just said, "Yeah." And I never went back to see a doctor again.

I just kept it—oh, I think I kept a lot hidden, because ... people were talking. But nobody really knew if I was pregnant or not. And to me, I just put it far back in my mind. I didn't tell nobody, I didn't tell nobody at all, there was only one person who knew about it—she was a good friend of my mother's, and she never told.

And then, one day I just started having pains, and they started hurting and I really thought that it was a stomach ache, I really did. And my mother, I told my mother I had a stomach ache and she was giving me all kinds of medicine to help the pain. It was Thursday night, I'd gone to school and I came home and the pain started. And then Friday morning I couldn't take the pain no more, I just couldn't, and I didn't know what it was, it was just that I felt that I had to go to the bathroom and I couldn't go. And then, I just went into the bathroom and I pushed, and the water bag didn't bust but it bulged out.

So then, my mom and me, this was about six in the morning, Friday morning, and me and my mother went walking to the hospital. And then, we got about halfway there and I couldn't walk no more and so I called up Ben, which was my boyfriend at the time, the father of the baby, and he came and we went to the hospital. And he didn't know either, you know, he didn't know, because I had lied to him too, I told him that I was taking the pill and he didn't know ... I was so young, and innocent, and I told him, you know, I just told him, "I'm going to have a baby." Then I got to the hospital at six-fifteen, and Benny was born at six-thirty.

The extreme to which the denial factor can be carried during pregnancy is illustrated by the following account of a girl who gave birth to her first child at the age of fifteen in her own home, with no one to assist her.

I had the baby here by myself. I know that's hard to believe, but I had him, I had him here.

Did your family know you were pregnant?

No! I hid it every possible way I could, because I was scared.

You carried it for nine months and nobody knew?

Nobody. I kept on saying, you know, putting this mental block in my head, "I'm not pregnant, I'm just gaining weight. I'm not—I'm just gaining weight—that's all I am." And I was not drinking. I drank a lot before I conceived, and I thought, "Well, it's just beer belly, it's just a beer belly." But one night my water broke, and I went all that day and then that night. I didn't feel nothing. I didn't really feel nothing. My mom and dad had gone away for the weekend. My sister was here, but she didn't know nothing. See, here I am, having labor pains, and it went for ten hours straight until about ten-five the next morning when I had him.

Were you in bed when you gave birth?

I was on the bathroom floor.

On the bathroom floor?

Yes.

You must have known what was happening?

Oh, yes!

But you had no help from anyone delivering your child?

No ... see, my sister, I yelled, "Connie!" I said, "Connie! Come here!" And she goes, "Oh, my God!" And she goes and calls the ambulance, and then the paramedics came and they took me to the hospital, and they stitched me up and got me back to normal.

I knew I was pregnant all this time. I knew it. But in the back of my head I'm saying, "No! No!—I'm *not!*"

CHAPTER THREE

Reactions to the Pregnancy

Once pregnancy had become an acknowledged fact, each girl was faced by the necessity of making a big decision. What should she do—have an abortion, give the child up for adoption, marry the father of the baby, or keep the child herself?

Some of the girls said that they were sure of what they wanted to do very early in their pregnancy. Others went through long periods of confusion and indecision. Some started to follow one plan, and then changed their minds.

Sooner or later, however, all but a few came to the realization that certain important people had to be taken into consideration. It wasn't enough just to talk over ideas with their friends. Their parents, the baby's father, and his parents—all would have strong feelings about what was happening, and would have to be told.

Except for six who had been married at an early age, the girls were unmarried when they became pregnant, and all but one of the unmarried girls were under eighteen years of age. In other words, they were legally minor children, subject to their parents' supervision and control, just as surely as they were dependent on them for food and a roof over their heads. Becoming pregnant did not give them instant adult status, it did not emancipate them from their parents; but it did create an unusual situation in which they actually had the last word—for a pregnant woman, whether she is forty or fourteen, has the right to decide what she will do about the pregnancy.

Many parents find this concept difficult to understand. They have always made the decisions affecting their children's welfare—why shouldn't they decide what should be done when a daughter becomes pregnant? "She is only a child," they say, "what does she know about raising kids?"

The stage is set for a highly emotional struggle, in which feelings based on years of living together get all mixed up with new feelings of disappointment, guilt, frustration, and anxiety, as parents and daughter struggle with a problem that has to be solved within a limited time.

In most cases the girls were well aware of what would happen when their parents got the news. Even figuring out how to tell them was so difficult that they put it off as long as possible. Janet's story is a good illustration of this. She had been unable to tell her parents she was pregnant, but a girl friend in whom she had confided eventually admitted the truth to Janet's mother, and then told Janet what she had done.

She said, "Your mom's here, she knows you're pregnant, and she wants to talk to you." And I said, "Dear God, you've got to be kidding," but I was sort of relieved when I knew that she knew.

My mom came to pick me up from school and we went over to my grandparents' house, and we had a really good talk. My mom told me, she said, "It's not the end of the world," and she was really understanding and it made me feel good. I felt more grown up when I was talking to her. She knew I smoked, but that was the first time I ever smoked in front of her. I said, "Do you mind if I have a cigarette?" I was so nervous.

But my dad, he was on a business trip, and the night that he came home I was so nervous, I just knew I couldn't keep it from him. I had to tell him, I just had to. I told my mom, when he came home I had to tell him because it was bugging me so bad, and I was so nervous I couldn't have gone to sleep that night.

So he took a shower and came in and I said, "I got to talk to you. Why don't you sit down?" He says, "Okay." And I told him. There's no way of going around telling somebody you're pregnant. I sat there and thought and thought and thought of some way to go around saying I was pregnant. Finally I just had to come out and say, "I'm pregnant." And my dad just cried, and I cried, and my mom cried. But then five minutes later he went up to Peter's house and I thought he was going to kill him. I was scared.

It was evident from several accounts that the announcement of pregnancy precipitated a major family crisis. Alison's story about the day she broke the news of her pregnancy to her parents captures the tension of the precise moment in which she realized that life for her and her parents could never be the same again.

I was living at my aunt and uncle's at the time I found out I was pregnant. It really broke my aunt's heart when she found out I was. She thought I'd let her down. And that didn't encourage me too much to feeling too good.

So finally the day I told my parents, I thought it was going to be a whiz, it would be so easy. Because I was mad at them at the time, I was rebellious, and so when I told them, or when I was thinking about telling them, I thought, "Well, this will just stick them." So, when we got there, I was sitting there, and I just couldn't say anything. And all my true feelings really started coming about. I never felt ashamed for being pregnant until the minute I told them I was. I could barely talk, I was fighting to keep the tears away, because I didn't want them to see how much I cared what they thought. And I had this huge lump in my throat that hurt *so bad*, and when I told them, my dad just started hitting his palm with his hand, and my mother was just smoking away on her cigarette and they … I was surprised. I thought for sure they'd jump and say, "Well, you're going to get an abortion." But they didn't. They asked me what I was going to do. And if Sam and I were going to get married, and what was going to happen. And the only negative thing that they told me is that I'd never move home again.

Hurt and shame were the parental reactions most dreaded, and most frequently experienced. Many girls referred to their mothers' anguish, tears, and emotional outbursts when they heard the news of the pregnancy; but somehow, the most touching of all the accounts of family reactions were those describing the feelings of fathers or brothers.

The hard thing was telling my dad. And when we told my dad, I think he was ashamed of me like, because he was so hurt to find out that I was pregnant, and he wanted to have nothing to do with me. Absolutely nothing.

In the beginning, when he found out I was pregnant, he said we would have to give it up for adoption because I was too far along to have an abortion. The first few nights it was hard. I could hear him arguing with my mom, and my older sister. They'd sit around and say what they were going to do with me and this baby. And then finally, after a few weeks had gone by and they had talked with my doctor and stuff, then my mom decided that the best thing for them to do was to go along with what I wanted. So they told me that. And I told them that I couldn't give it up for adoption. I couldn't do it.

But oh, I remember my dad! I was so afraid for him to see me big and pregnant, I used to kind of hide. I was still in my levi's and everything because I wasn't very big, but when I'd go by him, I'd try to hold my stomach in and try to hide it from him. And when I'd sew my baby stuff ... I never had a baby shower because my dad felt this wasn't right, but I'd still get a lot of things from friends. He didn't want me to go to the store. He wanted to keep me hid, I think, because he was ashamed and hurt.

When I started showing, I remember I was opening the garage door and that's the first day that my dad realized that I was pregnant and I was his daughter and he didn't need to treat me the way he was. I went to open the garage door and he came out and said, "Oh, you can't do that." That's when I felt better because my dad was finally opening up and being nicer to me. And then I remember when I was in my ninth month, and it was getting closer to the time, he had a surprise for me. He made a cradle, which I have pictures of now. My sister's using it now. He made me a cradle for the baby. And that was very touching when he did that.

In the story which follows, Jenny describes her brother's reaction when he got the news she was pregnant.

My older brother had just bought a house, and he came over one day to get some of his stuff that he'd left in his closet, and I was in here in my room. My mom and dad both decided they had better tell him, because I'd found out maybe a couple of weeks before. They didn't know how to tell him, they didn't know how he was going to take it. So they just both went in there, and they closed the door, and they told him. His room is right across from mine and I had my door open, so I was wondering what they were doing in there for so long.

He came out with tears in his eyes and said, "Jenny, come here," and he was just so shook up and so hurt he couldn't ... My mom told me that when he found out, well, the first thing he did was hit the wall, and then he just broke down crying. He didn't know if he should go and kill Stan, or if he should just sit and cry. So he called me and at first he just started yelling, he goes, "Don't you know how you get pregnant?" and stuff, and then he sat down and he just goes, "Well, I love you. You're my sister. And I just don't want this to happen to you."

Just as family reactions were extremely important, so was the boy friend's attitude, which varied, as might be expected, from sheer joy to outright rejection. The *quality* of the relationship between boy and girl, and the degree of commitment to each other, were the most important factors.

The boys were usually the same age as the girls or a little older; occasionally they were younger, even as young as fourteen or fifteen. Some were fully employed, others were going to high school, while still others were of school age but had dropped out.

A few stories will indicate certain reactions frequently encountered, and the effect they had upon the girls. Since a girl's parents were apt to be angry and critical of her when told about the pregnancy, she often turned to her boy friend for comfort. His feelings assumed enormous importance in her eyes and played an important part in the decision making process.

Sometimes the boy let the girl down completely, at the very time when she needed him most. For example, when Marjorie was returning home after a trip to the doctor's, she was both excited and also somewhat alarmed. She wanted more than anything else to talk to her boy friend.

The phone kept ringing and ringing and his mom finally answered. I asked to talk to Phil, and he got on the phone and I said, "Phil?" And he said, "What do you want?" I said, "You're going to be a father." And I don't remember quite the words that he said, but he put me down about it like he didn't want nothing to do with it and that upset me, you know. Well, it upset me because I was pregnant and I knew for sure. I'd heard the heartbeat and that really kind of scared me, having somebody else inside of me. I was trying to tell him about this, and he was just being a snot over the whole thing.

Probably a show of *some* emotion—even anger or recrimination—would have been preferable to a reaction devoid of any noticeable feeling, such as this girl experienced.

I think what bothered me the most was he never reacted. You know, I always thought he cared about me and stuff, but then when I would tell him, "Hank, I think I might be pregnant," he never said to me, "Well, if you are, we'll do this . . ." He just always said, "Well, you can't be."

When the pregnant girl is fifteen, and her boy friend is only fourteen, their ability to plan realistically has severe limitations.

My mother wanted me not to keep it. She wanted me to get an abortion, but the baby's father didn't want me to. "Well, you know," I thought to myself, "it's not going to be no trouble. It's going to be a baby and hardly no responsibility."

My mother was crying, she was hurt, she stopped me from seeing the baby's father until the time the baby was born. But I used to see him in school and stuff, so it really didn't matter. He didn't go to school, and he used to come to my school—he is eleven months younger than I am. So . . . we really weren't ready for a baby, we just thought we were, you know.

Every now and then a girl had the courage to point out to a boy that he too had a bit of responsibility as far as her pregnancy was concerned.

I told my boy friend, and at first he was excited and said, "Oh, that's neat." Then I think he got to panic after a while, and he said, "Well, what are you going to do?" And I said, "What am *I* going to do? We're in this together!"

Some boys, when faced by the news of the pregnancy, told the girls quite frankly that they were not ready to become fathers or to assume any parental obligation. First Marcia describes how her boy friend reacted.

He said he wasn't ready to have a baby yet and he wasn't ready to settle down, and that if I wanted to I could, but he wouldn't be around if I ever had a kid. And so then I didn't believe him, but then I had the baby and he just didn't come around no more.

Then Sheila tells how she felt about the pregnancy, and how her boy friend reacted.

When I first found out, I was young then, I thought it would go away. I didn't think something like that could happen to me, I guess I thought that I was too good—I don't know. When I told the father of my child, he said that he would think it over for a weekend, and he came back and said he couldn't handle it—he could handle me, but he couldn't handle the baby. So I didn't see him for about five, six months till the baby was born. And I thought he was going to stay with me—he made me believe it, he was talking to me about the baby, how much he loved it and everything. And, he came home with me, held the baby, and didn't come back. I haven't seen him since.

In contrast to the reactions of fathers so far described was the happy, supportive response of those young men who genuinely rejoiced at the news of the pregnancy. They had certain characteristics in common: a real affection for the girl, and a sincere interest in becoming a father. Usually they wanted to make immediate plans to get married, and accepted their obligation to support a wife and child. This is a big order, and sometimes, as in the following story, the young man was only seventeen.

Ken is a very emotional person—very, very emotional. But he's a man, and he's got this big hang-up, that he's the man and whatever he says goes. So you can imagine what kind of reaction he took towards it. He was so happy that he got a grin on his face from one side to the other! And yet, he was so nervous at the same time.

His first reaction—he just lit up, his whole face was just so happy, and he comes over and he grabs me and hugs me real tight and tears come to his eyes, and he says, "Oh, baby, you're pregnant! We're going to have a baby! You and me!" And he's squishing me real hard, because he's kind of a big man, and then he goes, "Oh, I'm sorry!" And he sits down and tries to hold my stomach, and he says, "Oh, baby!" and he's hugging me and stuff.

The reactions of the boy's family and the girl's family were often similar, although as one girl very shrewdly pointed out, there is a subtle difference.

His parents, they were shocked, but they didn't take it bad at all. They took it better than my parents did. I think it's probably because they've got a son—a son's different, I think, than a daughter.

Occasionally, on hearing the news of the girl's pregnancy, the boy's family took prompt and drastic action.

My mom and dad called his mom and dad, and they told them. Steve and I weren't there. I don't remember exactly what went on, but then they moved right away.

On the other hand, there were times when the boy's family showed tolerance and understanding which the girl felt were lacking in her own family.

None of them said, "Have her get an abortion"—not one of them. They said about marrying me, "Well, we just want you to be sure. We'll do anything we can to help you." They were just the opposite of my parents—I'll put it that way. They

were really understanding. You see, I told Fred's mother
before I told my own mother. I didn't have the face to tell my
mother. Now Fred's mother I could tell, because I knew that
she wouldn't come back at me like my mom would.

Fred's mom has helped us a lot. Fred's dad has helped
us—as much as you can think!—all our furniture here, our
table in the dining room, our chair, our couch, all that stuff he's
given us. So it's really great.

No matter what the final outcome was, the toughest job a girl
had to face was breaking the news of her pregnancy to all the
important people in her life, and if her boy friend was taking his
share of the burden, he suffered with her. Corinne's story begins
as she and her boy friend undertake the task of telling his parents.

So we went to tell my boy friend's mother. He was really—he
was so scared, because he comes from a very strict family—they're hard on their kids. Well, the father is. And that's
what he was afraid of. He really thought his father was going to
beat him something bad. He saw us coming, and he knew my
mom was going to tell his mother, so he took off. That's how
scared he was— he was so scared. And I waited. My mom told
his mother, and my mother was mad. His mother, she took
it really good. She was happy in a way, but she was dis-
appointed, but there was nothing she could do about it. So
then I waited for him to come back.

He was just gone for about an hour and he was really upset.
He was crying and the whole bit. He didn't know what to
expect out of his father. But his mother told his father, and she
told him kind of in a bad way, because she told him in front of
everybody. His father said, "Well, I guess that's it. You ruined
your life right there." He was in the tenth grade. "You're going
to have to quit school and get a job and support that baby." So
that's what he's been doing ever since then—working with his
dad and that kind of thing.

I lived at home and he lived at his house, because I
was only fifteen. I was fourteen when I got pregnant, but I was
fifteen when I had the baby.

CHAPTER FOUR

Attitudes toward Abortion

The atmosphere of tension and hurt feelings which often surrounded a girl, once her pregnancy became known, made it next to impossible for her to consider calmly and carefully the various alternatives open to her. She got lots of advice, lots of pressure—usually based on how other people felt about her being pregnant, and what it would do to *their* lives as well as hers.

Decision making regarding an unplanned pregnancy is rarely achieved through a cool intellectual process. When it involves an unmarried girl under eighteen years of age, problems often reach crisis proportions. The girl herself has strong feelings, which may include fear, guilt, anxiety, bitterness; powerful emotions, particularly the maternal urge; and grave doubts as to her own ability to take on a long-term responsibility she is not prepared for. Then come the intense pressures from parents, boy friend, family members, and friends. Opinions often differ. To accede to the wishes of the most insistent may represent a loss of personal identity, to oppose them usually exacts a high price.

Of the four possible alternatives—abortion, adoption, marriage, keeping the child—not one is altogether "right." On the contrary, each decision is apt to seem "wrong" to somebody important, in some aspect, or to some degree; hence it was of great interest to me to learn as much as possible about the girls' attitudes toward the various alternatives, and how they resolved the problem of decision making.

To be sure, all except one of the girls did ultimately keep their babies. But did they seriously weigh all the other alternatives, eventually discarding them one by one? What were their attitudes toward them? Did they "choose" to keep the baby because they wanted a child, *right then?* Or did they perhaps drift into this way of thinking because they couldn't accept any other?

Since the only one of the four alternatives that has any time limitations is abortion, this subject will be considered first. Abortion has been legal in California since 1967, but until the early seventies an abortion was difficult to obtain because of the complex restrictions imposed by the State Legislature. Gradually these were greatly modified in practice, and by the time the girls who were interviewed had become pregnant, abortion was a clearly available option.

It was not necessary to go to Los Angeles, for several communities in the areas where the girls lived provided safe abortion services. Of course, not everyone knew this. As one girl said, "I believed that the nearest place for an abortion was a million miles away, yet I find out that it's right nearby."

There was no real financial barrier to obtaining an abortion; if a girl or her family could not pay for it, application could be made for Medi-Cal (the California term for Medicaid—public funds). Again, this information was not always known, especially to someone just fourteen years of age, like the girl who remarked: "Well, I wanted to get an abortion, but I couldn't afford it, and I didn't know that welfare would pay for it."

There were, as there always are, important time factors involved: abortions are relatively simple if performed during the first three months of pregnancy, but as each week goes by after that, the complexity, the risk, and the emotional distress increase.

Did these young mothers, then, seriously consider abortion as a possible choice?

Many dismissed the subject with a flat statement, such as, "I don't believe in abortions," "I couldn't do that," or "That's not for me." A few elaborated on these thoughts.

I really did want to keep the baby, because I knew if I had an abortion I would have had to live with it the rest of my life. Even if I got married to someone else, I would have always remembered, and I would have always wondered if it was a boy or a girl, and what it would have looked like, and every time I saw another baby I'd probably start crying or something, because I think abortions are awful.

Others went so far as to say abortion is the same thing as murder.

I was really considering abortion, but I was scared to death because I don't believe in abortion—to me it's murder. But I don't care—they say under three months it's not murder because it's not a living thing. That's ridiculous, the baby is growing. If it wasn't alive it wouldn't be growing, you know. It's just murder, and I don't believe in it.

Still others based their opposition to abortion on religious grounds. The stand taken by the Catholic church against abortion is well known, and needs no documentation here. It is interesting, however, to note the rationale expressed by a girl who had been reared in a different faith.

I thought about abortion, but since I'm Mormon and I've always been brought up thinking that abortion is bad and you're killing somebody (I'm not really into the church that much, but it's a *nice* religion, I like it), I thought, "What if... what if they're *right*? And I did have an abortion and I killed something?" I don't think I ... it would have bothered me.

Closely related to religious feelings were those which were rooted in conscience, a deep sense of personal responsibility for one's actions.

A lot of people think that I should have got an abortion, but I just feel like it's my fault, and I shouldn't take that out on the baby. I knew the consequences, I knew what could happen, and it was no one's fault but my own, and I wasn't going to take that out on the baby.

Occasionally a girl expressed a willingness to condone abortion for others, while ruling it out for herself. Like Evelyn, who made this reply when I asked if she had seriously considered abortion.

Yes, I thought about it, I thought about it. I just couldn't bring myself to do it. I believe in abortions, but ... for my friends, I give them advice: "You're so young, you ought to go have an abortion." But when it came down to me having an abortion, I just couldn't really bring myself to do it. I was thinking, "This is my baby, and I got into this. I'm going to take responsibility for it. I'm just going to have my baby."

The following conversation with Trudy is "one of a kind," for she was the only girl interviewed who said that if she had it all to do over again she would have acted quite differently.

My first reaction was, I was very happy that I was pregnant. I thought it was going to be a bed of roses and I was going to be a mother and it was just the best thing in the world. However, if I had it to do all over again, I wouldn't.
You wouldn't what?
I wouldn't have had my child. I would have had an abortion.
Was an abortion possible for you?
Yeah. Well, it was. I found out I was pregnant when I was four months pregnant. So I had two weeks, and I didn't even think about an abortion at that time. I was just going to have my baby, and that's the way it is.

Although the girls had strong feelings of their own regarding abortion, they could seldom avoid being influenced by other people's attitudes. It is appropriate, therefore, to take a look at a number of situations in which girls describe how people who were very important to them felt about abortion, and what they advised them to do. Of course, if parents and boy friend supported their viewpoint, then there was no conflict, and planning appropriate to the decision could proceed. What interested me most were the situations where points of view decidedly differed.

Many boy friends were described as having strong feelings about abortion, for or against. When their attitudes differed from those of the girls, and they were willing to talk things out, some thoughtful discussions took place, as illustrated in the following comments.

1 I myself, when I found out I was pregnant, I was considering an abortion, because I thought I was too young and wouldn't be able to handle it. He said no, he wouldn't let me kill the baby, and in many ways, he said, having a kid wasn't all that bad.

2 Well, see, I had always been against abortion—fully. I thought it was rotten. But then, when it came down to *me*, I decided ... well, I don't know. I don't know if I can have a baby right now. And Bryan didn't want to get rid of it at all. He really was strongly for keeping it. So he talked to me, and we sat down and had long discussions, many of them, and we just decided that deep down inside that was what we really wanted, we thought we could make it.

The two couples just referred to had contemplated marriage, and did eventually go ahead with those plans. There was more insecurity in the situations described by two other girls.

1 He asked me how I felt about abortion, and I told him that it was fine for someone else, but I couldn't do it myself. And he said, "What if I asked you, because you know I love you, and we are going to stay together and everything?" And he goes, "But just right now, at this time in our lives, we don't need a child to start things out." And I asked him to please don't ask me, because I couldn't do it. And he said, "Okay, we'll work it out another way."

2 Then I talked to my boy friend about it. But him being young and all, he was just as young as I was, so he didn't know what to do hisself. So he thought maybe I should get rid of it, and I didn't think so. So that caused a big confusion right there. So I just went on and kept it. It was *hard*, but him, after a while he said it wasn't his baby ... and I was too far along to get rid of it then, so I just went on and kept it.

The following passage shows the limits to which a frightened boy can try to push his girl friend.

> He calls me about two days later, and he goes, "Stacy, we're going to ditch school Monday or Tuesday," and I said, "How come?" He said, "We've got to get you down to L.A." And I go, "For what?" And he goes, "Well, I found a lady down there that does an abortion for five dollars." And I go, "*What?*" I said, "Jeff, if I decide upon an abortion, I can get it here, you know. I can get it up here, I can get it in a hospital, the whole bit." He said, "What kind of abortion? There's a lady that does it with a hanger." And I said, "Jeff, you've got to be kidding! Don't you realize that's an old way that could kill me as well as kill the baby?" And he goes, "We can't let everybody know."

The most prolonged struggle and the greatest anguish, however, were reserved for those situations where serious conflict developed between these very young girls and their own parents. Often parents were kept in the dark until very late in the pregnancy, which intensified their anxiety and their feelings of anger, disappointment, or shame. For some, their daughter's plight brought back painful memories of their own early years as parents—experiences they had wanted their children to avoid. Many were still young themselves—in their mid-thirties—and just beginning to feel that they might start a new life of their own, now that the years of caring for young children were behind them. And then—the news that a teen-age daughter was pregnant!

Abortion, from a parent's point of view, often seems to provide the only solution which allows family life to proceed with as little interruption as possible.

> When my parents found out, they said we should just "go get an abortion, and that will be all, it will be like nothing ever happened, and you won't have to tell anybody or anything."

That simplistic approach is rarely effective, for it ignores the big problem of what happens when a girl insists on carrying out her decision, resisting all efforts of her parents to change her mind. The ensuing conflict is a curious one, and often long and bitter. The parents not only have their traditional authority to fall back on, but they also have a host of reasonable arguments to support their belief that abortion provides the only sensible solution. The young girl is apt to base her case mostly on her feelings, on her sense of right and wrong, on her confidence that she can do whatever she has to do—without having formed any clear-cut plan of how she will do it. She also holds a "trump card," so to speak, for she has the final say about whether or not to continue her pregnancy. A conflict of this sort is a major family crisis with enormous implications, certainly best described by those who have experienced it.

Audrey had recently turned fifteen when she learned she was two months pregnant.

> I was going to have an abortion. I had an appointment to have it, but I didn't go. I decided that I was going to keep the baby, so I didn't go.
>
> My mom and dad fought with me, they didn't want me to have my child. They kept on telling me to have an abortion, and kept on telling me and telling me, and I told them, "No, no, no," and they said they'd buy me anything I want, and I told them, "No, I don't want anything. I want the baby."

When Eileen's family learned that she was five months pregnant by a married man, a bitter family conflict erupted over the issue of abortion, with both parents insisting it was the only solution.

> I didn't think anything bad about it. All I knew is that I was in love with this guy and I was having something that was his and that was good enough for me. My mom said, "Don't you understand? He doesn't belong to you. What are you going to do when the baby asks you where his dad is—that he was married when you had him? You have to think about all of these things."
>
> Then she told me that she wanted me to get rid of it. And I said that I wasn't going to. She took me to a doctor and this doctor was going to give me an abortion. It was going to cost

them five hundred dollars. I was almost five months along, and I would have a saline. They kept saying, "You're going to get it." The first thing my dad said when my mom told him I was pregnant was, "No, she can't have it. She has to have an abortion and that's what she's going to have. I don't care how much it costs, she's going to have an abortion. What's my family going to say? What are my brothers going to say? Oh, man!"

I knew what I wanted to do already, and I had my mind made up. So they took me, and the only way I could get the abortion is if I said I wanted it. I told the man, "I'm not going to have it, and you can't make me have it." He said, "Well, you're right." He told my parents, "We can't give it to her unless she wants it." My dad got mad, he just walked out, all mad. All the way home I heard it, "Why didn't you get it? You made us look like a fool. We made all these arrangements for you, took the money out of the bank, you went in there and just made a fool out of us." I said, "I told you I wasn't going to have it."

So for about three months I didn't talk to them much and they didn't talk to me, because they were hurt.

Sometimes the boy friend's family brought extraordinary pressure to bear upon a girl. For example, Eva and her boy friend had decided to get married, after the pregnancy was discovered. Then the following incident occurred.

His mom was really upset, because we were young and we wanted to get married. She kept calling me and telling me, "I don't think he wants to marry you."

Then one day his mother called my mother and told her, "We'll have a meeting. I want to talk to you tomorrow morning." My mom told me and I said, "I wonder what she wants." So my mom went to the meeting the next day, just her and Raymond's mom, and she gave my mom fifty dollars for me to get an abortion.

I was so hurt that I went to her house that day and I just got the money and I threw it at her, and I said, "I don't need your son!"

Then Raymond tried calling me the next day, and I wouldn't talk to him. That was my mistake—I should have just let it out and told him, you know, what his mother had done. He didn't know what was wrong with me, so finally my mother told him that his mother gave me the money to have an abortion. He was really upset with her, and said that it was his baby and he wants it, and she's not going to stop us. And that was it. She never said anything more.

Of special interest were accounts of parents' efforts to get their daughters to have abortions despite the parents' own religious convictions. In the following case there had been no undue pressure, rather just a suggestion on the mother's part.

When I told my mom, the first thing she said was to get an abortion. I said, "Okay." So I went to the welfare office, I got everything set, all the papers and everything, on Friday. Monday morning at six o'clock I was supposed to go in to get the abortion, and I just … over the weekend I just kind of chickened out.
You say your mother suggested abortion?
Right away. It's the first thing that came out of her mouth.
And she's Catholic?
Uh-huh.
How do you reconcile that?
I don't know. Like I said, we're church-goers, but I guess maybe she thought it was the best thing for her daughter, you know. She didn't want her daughter to have to hassle with a kid, Catholic or no Catholic.

It is important to note that although the girls I interviewed were as a whole opposed to abortion, at one time or another some of them had tried to get abortions, and others had actually had abortions. This information usually came to the surface when we were discussing any other pregnancies they might have had in addition to the one which had resulted in the birth of the child (or children) listed when they volunteered to be interviewed.

Five reported having had abortions, and another had planned to have an abortion but had a miscarriage, *before* the birth of the first child. Reasons cited were their extreme youth (fourteen to sixteen years), and their unwillingness to let their parents know they were pregnant.

Six had had an abortion *after* the birth of the first child, another had planned to do so but had a miscarriage, and still another had requested an abortion but was refused by her doctor. Reasons for termination included possible damage to the fetus, ill health of the mother, and an unwillingness to bear an additional child at that particular time.

Occasionally, as an interview was drawing to a close, we would return to the general subject of decision making, and a girl would express some thoughts which had grown out of her experience.

Barbara's baby was just four months old at the time of our interview. I asked her whether she had considered any solution other than keeping the baby, whether she had given any consideration to terminating the pregnancy.

My mother wanted me to — to tell you the truth, she did. She told me that I was going to ruin my life, that I was going to ruin it for me and the baby's father. She said, "You're too young, you should wait." She's not just saying, you know, like a nagging mother. She's just saying it because she cares for both of us, she doesn't want to see either one of us unhappy.

Before I got pregnant, I always thought that's awful for someone to have an abortion. But I think that it's all right for someone that really can't take a baby, because sometimes I feel like I can't take the life that I have right now, because a baby is a lot of work. And there is going to be a lot more problems ahead of me, and I didn't really think I was going to be able to cope with all these things that are all going to hit me at once.

Angela's child was two and a half years old. I asked her whether she had strong feelings about abortion. Was it altogether wrong, or all right in certain circumstances?

I think it's the situation you're in. Like me ... if I were to get pregnant — which I'm very careful, I don't want to get pregnant — but if I were to get pregnant, I would either have to make up my mind to keep it and get married and stay home and take care of the kids — that's how it would be. Or ... either to get an abortion and go on as I've been. And it would be a very hard decision for me. I won't know what to do.

And I don't want to make another mistake. I want to be sure. I want to *know* I want this baby — be prepared for it, you know, be married, have a house. I really want to have a house before I have any other — you know, have a home for my child, not be moving from an apartment to another place.

CHAPTER FIVE

Attitudes toward Adoption

Until the late sixties, continuing the pregnancy and giving the child up for adoption was the solution frequently chosen in cases of out-of-wedlock pregnancy, especially if the girl involved was white and from a middle class family. Adoption was not favored widely by black or Mexican-American girls. By the early seventies, however, as abortions became increasingly available, those who might in earlier years have given their babies up for adoption were apt to choose abortion instead.

In view of the sharp decline in numbers of babies relinquished for adoption nation-wide, it seemed important to find out how the young mothers who were interviewed felt about adoption. How much serious consideration had they given to it?

The interviews produced a far greater volume of material on the subject of adoption than had been anticipated. Not only had four girls actually relinquished a child (three of these the result of a pregnancy preceding that of the child they kept), but a number of others had seriously considered adoption at one time or another. Thoughts regarding adoption from several points of view were brought out into the open. Some had been adopted themselves, and expressed their feelings about this. Others were considering whether or not to encourage a husband or boy friend to adopt a child of theirs that had been born out of wedlock. Still others expressed a desire to take additional children into their family eventually through the process of adoption.

As in the case of abortion, the idea of adoption often becomes a highly emotional subject. It, too, is a subject on which people are not likely to feel neutral, and members of the same family frequently have opposing views. But adoption is a much more tolerable concept, generally speaking, than abortion. It is rarely labeled as "wrong."

The real problem with relinquishing a child for adoption is the way in which it conflicts with the concept of possession. If a child "belongs" to a person, can he or she give it to anyone else? And this is no ordinary object that is possessed, but a child that has come from a woman's own body and is therefore often considered a part of herself. This is the way one young mother put it.

> Like me, I never considered adoption because once I had my little girl, she was already a part of me, you know. I loved her, right as soon as the minute she came out. I knew that I could never give her up, I mean, she's my own, I had her, she grew in me for nine months. I mean, you can't just give a child away like that. I thought, you know, she's mine, you know.

A decision to relinquish a child requires a high degree of maturity and unselfishness. This fact was perhaps not sufficiently recognized and dealt with in years past, when a young girl was sometimes swept into a decision to relinquish her child by the sheer momentum of her family's insistence, by the purposeful efforts of church or agency personnel, or by the professional pronouncements of doctors or lawyers. Current practice in reputable adoption agencies is to provide ample opportunity for both the young mothers and the young fathers to make thoughtful decisions, based on their own consideration of all the factors involved.

When a girl contemplates relinquishing a child for adoption, she faces a problem with no clear-cut answers. Whichever way she moves, there will be some sorrow, some sacrifice. If she gives the child up, she may live to regret it. If she keeps the child, she may eventually wish that she had given it up. This sixteen-year-old girl described the ambivalence which tormented her both before and after the birth of her child.

> When I was about seven or eight months, when no one knew yet, I didn't want to have her ... I wanted to have her and then give her up ... because if I would have did that nobody would have known. Like I could have just went and had her

and then left the same day like I did, and then nobody would have known that I gave her up. I was afraid, and I thought it would be best for her, because I wouldn't have to worry about being on welfare, and the person could give her a lot more than what I could give her ... Because it takes a lot out of you. I thought about it even after she was born, I was thinking about doing it. I just never did. Sometimes I want to and sometimes I don't. It's just like when she gets on my nerves—it's not really her, it's everybody, when they start yelling at me and stuff— that's when I can't stand it. That's when I think that it would be better if I gave her up.

Celeste at fourteen realized that adoption would solve problems she was not prepared to deal with, but she wanted her child. For a while she took refuge in day dreams.

I didn't want *him* off my hands, I wanted the *responsibilities* off my hands, the responsibilities of a whole new little life. I wanted it off my hands, but I wanted him because I loved him. I would have loved to have a live-in maid take care of him— and we'd love him, but she'd take care of him! I would have loved that! But that wasn't reality.

It often takes years to figure out what really motivated a specific action. Here Kay, at twenty, married and the mother of two, discusses why, in retrospect, she and the baby's father rejected the idea of adoption when they were both sixteen.

It's not so much what I went through, it's what my child went through. I know, I really know that he probably would have been better off if I had given him up for adoption in the first year or so. Now I feel like we've done as well as anybody else could have, but at first I felt very guilty that I kept him. I felt like I was just too selfish—it was, it was very selfish, because I thought—here we have no money, no home, just got married, in an apartment—and yet I knew I couldn't give him away. I knew, because it would break my heart too much. So I felt very guilty to keep him just for my own need.

Frank definitely did not want him given up for adoption. When I said, "What should I do? Should I give him up for adoption?" he said, "No way." He couldn't stand knowing that somewhere out there is his child, and somebody else is taking care of him. So we decided to make the best of it, and it worked out.

The importance of the attitude taken by the baby's father can not be overestimated, for it is a dominant factor in helping the girl make up her mind. Although the feeling expressed by Frank, that "somewhere out there is his child," occurs over and over in accounts of adoption, the emotional response in his case was backed up by a degree of maturity far greater than his age would suggest. He wanted to marry Kay, he felt sure he could support his family, and he was ready to assume responsibility.

By way of contrast, the following episode describes the initial reaction of a young boy who had not even known his girl friend was pregnant, when he heard the news that he was a father and that the girl had already made plans to relinquish the child for adoption.

I went to his house and we went in and sat down. He was being really mean to me. I said "Hi" and he said, "What do you want?" I was scared to tell him anyway, you know. So we sat down and I gave him the papers stating that the child was in a foster home. I showed them to him and he said, "What does this mean?" and I said, "It means I had a baby about a week ago." And he said ... well, I can't say what he said ... And after that, I told him the story and he said, "Are you sure you want to give him up for adoption?" and I said, "Yes. What else can we do? I'm fourteen, you're sixteen. What else can we do? We can't do nothing. Me and you don't get along, we can't get married, and even if we do, what could we give him?" So he said, "All right. I'll sign the papers. You're right. We can't really do that much for him."

Claudia's boy friend had a serious drinking problem. She was a realist, and sufficiently well informed about the rights of natural fathers to take this factor into consideration as she struggled to make a wise decision.

I thought about adoption. I thought about it seriously quite a few times. And I think the thing that maybe ... well, I would have kept her anyways, but it kind of helped me because they said the father has the right to take it if you don't want it. And if he would have taken it, then it would have been raised with a bunch of drunks. And I didn't want that.

The attitude of a young father sometimes undergoes changes as the pregnancy proceeds. Elaine was married young, and she and her husband had planned to postpone having a family until she had finished high school. But at the beginning of her senior year she discovered she was pregnant.

Before the baby was born my husband got bored with his job fast. It scared me to death, because my parents said, "Once you get married, that's it. He's responsible for you." And I thought, "Well, here's this kid that doesn't even know his own life, how's he gonna support me and our baby?" And I thought a lot in my own mind about abortion, but it was too late. So I had to think, "Okay. What if he leaves me? What am I gonna do?" And then I seriously thought about adoption. Very seriously.
But when we started La Maze classes, he started feeling more like, instead of just starting the whole pregnancy, he was a part of it. He began to feel that it was our baby and nobody else's baby, and that we were the ones meant to raise it.

No matter how the boy friends felt about adoption, parents were the ones most likely to exert real pressure on the girl—sometimes for, sometimes against adoption. This girl's parents left no room for doubt.

My parents wanted me to give the baby up. They had told me if I didn't get married I had to give the baby up. So they more or less gave me an ultimatum. It was one or the other.

The authoritative approach just described is more familiar, perhaps, than the reaction of parents who oppose relinquishment. Two examples of parental opposition present the dilemma faced by a girl who knows in her own heart she is not ready for a child and sees adoption as a way out, only to meet with formidable opposition from members of her own family.

First is the story of Carlotta, who was very unhappy about being pregnant at sixteen. At the time of the interview her little girl was two years old.

> My mom and everybody kept telling me, "No, you have to have it. You can't do away with a baby … give it away like a dog, you know." So I go, "No, I don't want it. I don't want the baby—especially if it's a little boy. If it's a little boy, I don't want it."
>
> I still resent her. I mean, I love her and everything, but I still resent her. Like when I want to go out or when I want to go on trips—I'm involved in a lot of things, I like to go places. I could have gone to San Francisco, but I couldn't because I didn't have a baby sitter, and so I was upset. And I don't know … I get mad, and I just push … I never hit her hard or anything, but I just push her … "Get outa here! Go in your room!" … because she don't listen to me.
>
> *Do you feel that your family talked you into keeping her?*
>
> Yeah, they did. Because if it wasn't for them, I would have given her up.

In the second instance, Ruth was dismayed at the idea of becoming a mother, and expressed these doubts to her parents along with her alternative proposal.

> I was kind of wondering, "How am I going to take care of it? I'm only fourteen, I can't get a job—most jobs you have to be sixteen." Made me think I'd better put the baby up for adoption. And then my dad said, "I'd never give my baby up for adoption, my own flesh and blood." And my mom started crying. That's what did it, and that's why I really kept her. I

just thought I'd go through life with all these voices pounding in my ears, that's what really did it.

But I said, "How am I going to support it? I haven't got a job, and I still have to graduate from school. I'm only fourteen, you know, and you expect me to be a parent, stay at home, take care of a baby." When you're fourteen, you want to go out, go bowling, anything. And they say, "We'll take care of her." But that was only when I was pregnant. After I had the baby—"Change her diaper! You can't go out—you have a baby to take care of! Do this! Do that! She's your baby!"—and all this stuff. So when you're pregnant, they tell you, "I'll take care of her, you won't have to do hardly anything, you'll be able to go out and everything," but then when you have her, "No, you got to stay home, it's your responsibility."

If I had it to do all over again, I don't really know if I'd do it the same way again. I'd think a lot more about adoption.

Some girls who have second thoughts about the wisdom of keeping a child decide to put their doubts to the test by going through a "trial separation." They surrender the baby to the care of someone else, either formally through the help of a social agency, or informally through friends. In the following passage Crystal, who had kept her child against the advice of parents and boy friend, tells how she felt after the first flush of excitement had faded and she began to suffer from "after baby blues."

When I had the baby, everybody was all excited. I had her on a Monday, and he came that night and he was all "Oh, I'm the father and I'm so proud" and everything. Three days later I came home from the hospital, and he'd bring his friends over and show her off. Then I didn't see him for about a month or so.

I went to live with a friend. I was taking care of her kids for her while she worked. Well, she had two kids, and I had my baby, which is a lot of pressure, and I was depressed because Walt left me, and all this kind of stuff, and it just got really bad and I sat down and I thought, "Wow! I have a kid. What am I going to do?" And so I thought, "This isn't fair. It's not fair to her and it's not fair to me." I really got to thinking and I go, "Well, I'll give the baby up for adoption."

I called a woman I know who said that she had someone that would take the baby and everything, and she arranged it the next day. Well, that was really sad, because I cried and cried ... I didn't have her for a month, and the people that had her were going to adopt her.

It was terrible—the way I felt! I should have never let her go in the first place. I really don't think that's what I wanted. I think that's what everybody else wanted for me and I was under the pressure, and I thought ... "Well, screw it, I'll do it and make everybody happy. Except for me." And I thought about it after she was gone for maybe two or three days, and I thought, "I'm gonna get my baby back. There's just no way I'm not gonna get her back!" And I thought, "Why should I care what anybody else thinks? Think about Crystal for once." And I did. I got her back and I'm really happy about it.

Hospital staff members and social workers from adoption agencies are often assigned to talk with young unmarried mothers soon after delivery, to see if they are receptive to the idea of relinquishing their babies for adoption. This is a very sensitive, emotional time for the young mother, and anyone who approaches her must be prepared for resistance. If authoritative tactics are used, she will often become angry and depressed. Speaking of the people who talked with her in the hospital one girl said, "They really make you feel rotten. They tell you, 'You can't handle it, you're only fifteen. You'd better give this baby away!'"

Another girl, just fourteen years old, had started adoption proceedings while in the hospital and allowed her baby to be placed in a foster home. Later on she changed her mind. This is her version of what happened.

The social workers from the adoption agencies, the main thing that they are paid to do is to talk you out of that baby as fast and as good as they can. Before the baby is an hour or older, they want to talk you out of that baby. I know this for a fact, because the social worker told me, "I was supposed to talk you out of it," but I was bound and determined to keep my baby. I was bound and determined to try, and I was bound and determined to do a good job. I convinced him, so he didn't try to take the baby away from me. They don't actually take it away from you, they talk you out of it. They say, "That kid's going to cry all day and all night, and you're going to want to go out," and they present all the bad sides of having a baby in exaggerated terms. He did it for a little while, he'd do it off and on, but more or less my social worker was behind me and he helped me keep the baby.

In contrast to the preceding stories of adoption plans half formed and then discarded, of proceedings started and abruptly stopped, there was one instance in which the complete process of adoption was handled very swiftly. It is the story of a girl who remembered vividly what had happened nearly three years before the day we talked, when she had relinquished a child for adoption. The whole process had gone like clockwork — but the wounds it caused had been left for time alone to heal.

The next day a hospital staff member came and she goes, "Would you like to put this baby up for adoption?" And I go, "Who said anything about adoption?" Then she goes, "Well, you don't have to if you don't want to."

Then I got to thinking, "What kind of a life could I give him?" And I started thinking and I started to cry.

There's this rooming-in policy at the hospital, and I go, "Why am I seeing him? Why am I changing diapers? Why am I doing this if I'm going to put him up for adoption? Why? Tell me." That baby stayed in my arms. Nothing could break us apart. If I ate, it was with him in my arms. And then the day came when I was ... the day came ...

Three weeks later I signed the final papers. And it took me two years, two years ... to get over that. Deep inside me I've wanted a child that I could love, that I could take care of. My little girl replaces Derek in a lot of ways. But it isn't Derek. Derek's going to be three his next birthday. I don't consider him a baby. In my mind I see him as a baby, but I say to myself, "He's almost three years old."

On the final papers I have—when he's eighteen, if he wants to find me, they damn right better let him, because I let my address and everything be known.

He's my—I can still consider him my son. No matter what happens, I still consider him my son ... no matter what, it's a piece of paper ... you know, nine months of living with him in my stomach. Nine months! And then that little piece of paper saying that he's not my son!

Whether or not to give up a child for adoption must be rated among the most agonizing of all possible decisions. Wise adoption workers recognize this, and spend a great deal of time with the mother both before *and after* the adoption, to insure that her emotional needs are met and her self esteem preserved intact. If the mother's needs are neglected, she may choose to grieve for a long period of time over her loss instead of viewing her action as a gift to her child, a chance for a better life than she could give him.

Two girls told stories that showed adoption in a positive light. The first story concerns a girl who had mentioned only one child when she volunteered to be interviewed. As we talked, however, she revealed that she had had an earlier child, and relinquished it for adoption when she was only fourteen.

Her father was in this area, but we didn't converse or anything. For that matter, he didn't even know my daughter was born until two weeks after she was born, and then he had written a letter saying, "I love you, don't give the baby up," this and that, you know—just a lot of b.s., if you ask me. And my mind had been made up. I had been hurt, I was confused, I didn't know what I was going to do. So, I gave my baby up for adoption.

Looking back at it now, in a way I wanted the baby because it gave me room to grow up a little bit. I was still very, very young, and I had been sheltered all my life. In a way, I wish that it had never happened. But I made the decision to give my baby, my first child, up for adoption for the simple reason I was very young, I had not finished my education, I didn't know what I wanted to do with my life. I wasn't even sure whether I could take care of a child properly. I still feel it was the best thing for me to do.

The second story illustrates how important it is for a young pregnant girl to have the understanding support of her parents. It shows how parents and others can help her to assess her total situation, and see her life in reasonable perspective. Only when she has done that is she able to decide whether she is ready to accept responsibility for a child.

Well, by the time I really went and found out, I was about four or four and a half months pregnant. I told my mom right away. She understood—I think she must have cried for three days in a row—but she understood. My dad was on a business trip at this time, so he didn't know until he got back and my mom told him. And he understood, too. They just tried to help me the best way they could. They said they would help me raise the baby. This is what my mom said. But my dad right from the start thought that I shouldn't keep it.

When I first heard adoption, I was horrified! Adoption! Because I always imagined adoption as—that the child was in some foster home waiting to find a parent. I didn't realize how many parents are waiting for babies.

My mom felt the same way I did when she heard adoption from my dad. She thought, "How could you do this? How could you say this?" She thought it was such a terrible thing. Then she talked to a priest about it and he told her, he goes, "How old is she?" She says, "Sixteen." He goes, "You know she is still a child herself. It's a child raising a child. It's not fair to either of them." He thought adoption would be the best thing, too.

The more I talked to people, I found out so many people—my friends, so many people I know—are adopted, that I had never known before. Then I started talking to the adoption workers and found out how long the list is of people just waiting for babies.

If I had thought that the best thing for my baby would have been for me to keep him, I would have. I would have done anything for him, because I just wanted him to have the best, and if I couldn't give it to him, then I wanted somebody else to. Here I was, a junior in high school, sixteen, planning to go to college, getting good grades and everything, then all of a sudden, *this* comes! I was ready to give that all up for him, but it just wouldn't be fair to him.

The one thing that bothered me so much when I gave him up for adoption was that I didn't want him to ever think that he wasn't loved or wasn't wanted. It was *because* he was so wanted that he was given up. So I wrote him a letter, and I wrote the parents a letter, and I gave them to the adoption worker to give to the parents; and a picture of me, too, to give to the baby when he starts getting old enough to want to know more about his parents. Because I know that if I was adopted I would want to know who I looked like, and I would want to know why I was given up.

I think it was good. I have grown up so much in the last nine months, and learned so much, that I'm just a totally different person. I think it *has* been good for me. It was a lot of pain, and a lot of heartache and hurt, but I have gotten a lot out of it. I've learned a lot. I've learned what I really want in a guy, and how I really feel about a lot of things, and what's really important to me. For a lot of people, it doesn't always come out that way, because they'll say, "Oh, I'll never have a baby again. I'll never go through that again." For me the whole thing of childbirth was just so great that I can't wait to get married and have a kid, and be able to keep him.

CHAPTER SIX

Marriage as a Solution

It is customary, when discussing the options available to a girl who is pregnant out of wedlock, to include marriage to the father of the baby as one of the "solutions." It could be argued that in reality there are only three possible alternatives, not four; that they are abortion, adoption, and keeping the child, and that marriage is merely a factor which separates those that keep the child into two groups: those who marry, and those who remain single.

Ideally, of course, marriage deserves to be considered solely on its own merits, without reference to a pregnancy or any other specific situation. But when pregnancy has occurred unexpectedly, the situation is not exactly ideal.

The use of the word "solution" as a synonym for "alternative" or "choice" when discussing decision making during pregnancy is significant. It implies that there is a "problem" which requires solving—in this case, a pregnancy which was unplanned, or even unwanted. There are only limited "solutions" available for this problem, and each one of them is anxiety producing, and may bring with it a whole new set of problems along with whatever advantages it offers.

Marriage is the time honored solution in cases of unplanned pregnancy. Before adoption and abortion were viable choices, a pregnant woman who did not marry had to be brave enough to raise an illegitimate child. Now, although the stigma attached to illegitimacy has been considerably reduced, the specter of it remains, especially in the minds of the generation which includes the parents of the girls who were interviewed. Marriage is still seen as the best way to "give the child a name," to assign responsibility for its support, and to obtain the blessing of the church and the respect of the community. To be sure, haste is imperative. Children are supposed to come *after* marriage, not before, but since pregnancy has ruled out that possibility, the next best thing is to make plans for a marriage as soon as possible.

The reasoning just described explains why marriage during pregnancy is often viewed as a "solution." As the girls discussed their own experiences, however, other attitudes regarding marriage were made very clear. Some had considered marriage but felt that being pregnant was not a valid reason in itself for marrying. As one said, "Marriage isn't based on a kid, it's based on love." In view of the fact, however, that 28 of the girls interviewed did get married during pregnancy — 15 of these during the first three months — we can not dismiss the concept of marriage as a "solution," nor can we assume it is irrelevant and outmoded.

Although 54 girls were married at the time they were interviewed, in this chapter only the experiences of the 28 who were married *during pregnancy* will be considered, for they are the only ones who can be said to have chosen marriage as a solution to the pregnancy.

It seemed important to learn from these girls what their experiences had been. What were the circumstances surrounding their decision to get married? How had their families reacted? What was the attitude of the father of the baby? How did the provisions of the 1970 California law regarding marriages of minors affect them?

The attitudes of the girl's parents and the boy's parents had a great deal to do with the ultimate success or failure of their plans to get married. These attitudes, as might be expected, varied greatly. In general, the weight of tradition, and the fear of criticism from relatives and friends, were factors which made parents look favorably on the idea of marriage. But they had their share of worries about the youth and immaturity of the young people, and their own feelings of hurt and frustration to deal with, and so there was many a tense situation. One father who was furious at the news of his daughter's pregnancy shouted: "I don't want to see her. I don't want to see him. Get them out of my house!" — and then gave them permission to be married.

In some instances a couple had been planning to marry

eventually, and the pregnancy just hastened their plans. In Shirley's case a great many important events were packed into a few days.

I found out that I was pregnant the first week of my senior year. And—well, everything was just really kind of fast, you know. I think I found out on Tuesday and I told my parents on Wednesday and we got married on Saturday!

I didn't know exactly what I was going to do. We had planned on getting married, but we were going to wait a couple of years, you know, we'd been going together for a year and a half. And I don't know, I was just kind of dumbfounded, I guess, I didn't know what to do.

Then I went over and talked to Tony about it. He was pretty shocked when he found out. I think he was scared. He was never mad, he was never mad about it, you know. The only thing was he had planned on going to college and stuff, you know, and it kind of messed that up. He tried to go for a while, but it just didn't work out, you know, later. But I think he was more scared than anything else, really. Because he wasn't very old either, he was only nineteen—I was seventeen and he was nineteen.

I told my mom the next morning—that's funny, too. I went in and told her, and I started crying, and she looks at me and she says, "Well, don't cry—there's nothing to be upset about." She just looks at me and she says, "You know, I should be mad at you, but I've been wanting a grandbaby for so long!" So, she wasn't really upset about it or anything, you know. My dad was, but she wasn't.

I didn't tell him—my mom did. And he didn't talk to me for a couple of days. Then him and Tony went out—I guess it was Friday—they went out, and they came in—they'd had a couple of drinks—and he comes in and he says, "I tried to be mad at you, but I just can't be mad. I love Tony like a son, you know, I couldn't ask for any better son-in-law." He says, "Okay, whatever you want to do, that goes. If you want to get married, you get married. If you don't want to get married, don't get married," he says. "It's up to you, it's totally up to you. Don't feel like you have to get married just because — you know, to save your reputation or to keep us from anything," he said. "If you want to have that baby," he said, "we'll be more than happy to pay your medical bills, to take care of you and the baby and everything." I said, "No, we want to get married." And he said, "Okay." He told Tony the same thing, you know, not to marry me just because he felt like he had to. It worked out really good.

We all went to Las Vegas. I kind of wanted to get married in a church, but we got married in a chapel and we had a regular minister and everything, and it was really nice. It was pretty, you know, we got the record and the pictures and everything. It was real nice. Then my parents had a big reception for us two weeks later. So it turned out really, really nice.

Some girls did not feel the kind of family support which Shirley enjoyed, and for them the decision to get married often involved a great many problems. For example, Sylvia and her boy friend had been planning for a long time to be married eventually, but when she became pregnant they put off even telling their parents about it because they were so afraid of their reaction. As she said, "Nobody had expected this of us. We were good students. It just was a thing that happened — it wasn't like I was a tramp or anything. And it really bothered me, I was so afraid my parents were going to think I was so rotten. And his, too." She finally told her parents when she was six months pregnant, and they *were* upset. But in three days time they went to Las Vegas — where more troubles awaited them.

His father didn't go with us to Vegas, he didn't want to have anything to do with it. His mother went, and my mother and father went, and we got it taken care of.

We were shanghaied by a lawyer there who ripped us off for something like $150 to get me married.

I'm not sure exactly what happened. We went in there and we didn't know where to go. We didn't know if we should go to a chapel, or if we should go directly to the justice of the peace. So we stopped at a wedding chapel. And the man said, "Well, just a minute." First of all he says, "Are you pregnant?" Just like that! And I went, "What do *you* think?" Anyway, he was a very disagreeable person, with an old cigar hanging out of his mouth. He called over to the courthouse, talked to some lady, and said, "Okay, I'm sending them over now." And he said, "Be sure you talk to so-and-so"—I don't remember the name right now.

So we went across the street and talked to this particular woman, and she said it was going to cost us $150 to have the lawyers write up a consent form, or something like that—some kind of a form—that that was how much it was going to cost to have the lawyer sign it. And I couldn't believe it, because nobody I'd ever talked to had said that. See, they knew our situation—this man must have known somebody over at the courthouse, and he sensed our situation and figured—well, here was somebody he could rip off. And he sure did, because there was nothing we could do about it. My dad wanted us married, and *we* wanted to get married—that part of this hurdle was solved. So we went over there and paid about $150. To get married!

Sometimes all but one of the four parents involved agree with the young couple's decision to get married, and yet the disapproval of that one is felt so keenly that it is as if a shadow were cast over any attempt to celebrate. In Sylvia's case it was her future father-in-law who showed his displeasure by refusing to go to Las Vegas with the others. In the story which follows, the tension created by the negative attitude of the groom's mother is painfully clear.

We wanted to get married in a Catholic church, so we had to talk to one of the priests privately, because it is more or less a sin in our church, you know, to have gotten pregnant before we got married. We went through all the classes, and his mother was still very—I don't know—she just really didn't want us to get married. She finally agreed to sign the papers.

And my father was overdoing it, trying to be nice, and it was just making a touchy situation, it was really tense. But they finally signed them.

Then my mother says, "You know, we made a date when you could be married." I was going to have my friend as maid of honor, and he was going to have his best friend. My grandmother and a few of my relatives were coming. So my mother called up his mother and says—well, first Jim called his mother and says, "Lisa's mother wants to have a little something, you know, a little cake and champagne, because this is going to be the only time we get married and we might as well have a little something out of it"—and she hung up. She said, "You know how I feel about it"—click! I got all upset and cried, and so my mother called up and said she'd try talking to her. She said, "You know, this is the only time the kids are going to get married, and it's not a big thing, but I thought you'd like to come, and I've invited Jim's aunt and I've invited my sisters and brothers, and I thought you'd like to come, too." She just kept saying, "No, no, Jim knows how I feel about it," and she hung up again.

So Jim felt bad, and he didn't want any of my friends to come, because he felt embarrassed that his parents weren't going to come. So my dad got on the phone to his dad, and his dad said, "Well, I'll try to change her mind, but I just don't think I can." It just got to be a real hassle—right down to the wire we didn't think they were coming. Jim told me, "I don't want any of your friends there," because he was embarrassed, and I saw how he felt. He felt, Guy! his parents wouldn't even come, and all his friends would come and say, "Hey! Where's your mom?" So I didn't tell my friends, but being as close as I have always been with friends, they showed up!

On the way home from the church, I see this little girl on the lawn, and I told Jim, "Gosh! doesn't that look like your little sister?" and he says, "Yeah!" and then we see his dad's truck. They showed up—don't ask me why—and there's never been a problem since. I walked in the door, and they hugged me and said, "Welcome to the family!" and everything was fine. We had a nice big party—champagne, beer keg, the whole bit! It was really nice.

There was a variety in attitudes toward marriage among the girls themselves. Some, by sheer determination and grit, had managed to make a success of a marriage that had started out under most discouraging circumstances. Penny, for instance, who had been married for six years at the time of the interview, said she had felt a lot of pressure from her parents, particularly her mother. "There was no way that she would let me keep the baby and not be married," she said. "She just told me that we get married or I go to one of these homes and give the baby up. So we got married." In answer to my question, "How did you feel about marriage?" she made this reply.

> I don't know. At the time I was kind of excited about it, you know. It was a new thing—I got to be away from my parents—I was kind of excited about it. Then after a year, I was kind of thinking, "What am I doing? I don't want to be married." My husband and I have never had any problems, but I was fifteen when we got married, and that's awfully young to settle down.
>
> When we got married, my mom wrote a letter that I found, and it said, like ... "within the year she'll be back home, we'll have to support the baby, her husband will be off somewhere and he won't support it." And I think ... when we had our roughest time, I think that's what kept us together. Because in a new marriage you always have problems, and this and that. But I kept thinking, "I'm going to show her I can do it." My sisters have been through divorces, and I keep thinking, "That's not going to happen to me." And I am so content now in my marriage that I can never see that in the future. Things always pop up, but I can't see that for us now.

Whereas Penny accepted her parents' ultimatum and set out to prove she could make a success of her marriage no matter what, Celia arrived at a decision to get married only after a long, painful struggle with her own conflicting feelings. Problems in her own family were becoming too much for her, and she longed to have a life of her own, but she worried for fear she might be marrying for the wrong reasons.

For his eighteenth birthday present, that's when I found out I was pregnant—on his birthday. So he had just turned eighteen and I was just sixteen. He wanted to get married right away, and I told him no, I didn't want to, because I didn't want a marriage that was just based on the fact that I was pregnant. But that was his idea completely. He says, "We're getting married. That's all there is to it. That's my baby, and we're getting married." And I said, "Well, if that's the way you feel, if you don't feel you're getting pushed into it, that's fine with me."

So we told our parents that we were getting married. The first three days—I remember, the first three days my mother was very understanding and very kind to me. We told her like I said, and at first she thought it was a joke. And I said, "No, it's the truth, I'm pregnant and we're getting married." She said, "We'll take you to Las Vegas and get you married." And I said that would be fine. And she said, "Well, I'm glad I was sitting down for that." I told her I didn't want to tell my dad because I thought sure he would just kill me. She just asked him if he wanted to go to Las Vegas to get me married and he said, "Fine." He said, "Those who play have to pay," and laughed it off.

I think it was the first three days that were the shock and they were able to be kind to me. After that, after it wore on, my father—he never said anything, he never said anything to me about it or to Dick. And there were other problems.

Finally it just got to be too much. I just wanted to get out of the whole family, because I had always been told that once you get married, that *that* is your family. You just break away from your parents and you start your whole new family yourself. So I think I really wanted that, I wanted a whole new life.

Dick didn't know just how serious the situation at my

home was, but he had a feeling and he said, "Is this why—are you marrying me because you love me, or because you just want to get away?" And I said, "Well, I'm going to be perfectly honest with you. I care a lot about you, that's why I'm pregnant, but the love, you know, we'll just have to wait and see about." Thank God that worked itself in! But I think that's kind of bad, too. You don't marry just because you're pregnant. You marry because you love him. I did fall in love—it didn't take long—but I think it would have been better if it had started before that, if I hadn't had all the little things that bothered me.

It was a real hostile time, everyone was on everyone's nerves, and no one was really looking forward to the baby, and instead of it being a happy time it was more of a depressing time for me. My first baby wasn't—I can't think of the word— I guess really *wanted*, at the time, you know. I wanted her and Dick wanted her, but no one else really wanted to accept the fact that she was on the way. But with my second child, everyone was so happy for me, you know, and it's like she's my first baby!

Sometimes a difference in religious background causes a great deal of anxiety and family friction. Irene and her boy friend thought they had worked out a compromise which recognized the rights of each, but like most compromises, it did not please everyone, and she suffered most of all.

See, that was one problem when we got married, because I'm Catholic and—well, we're all Christians—but he's a Baptist. And his parents used to be Catholics but they converted to this religion, and they're real religious, very religious. They don't smoke or drink or anything. So when we got married, my mother wanted us to get married in the Catholic church, and then his parents wanted us to get married in their church. So that's why we ended up getting married in Mexico first—so it wouldn't bring up any problems, you know.

Then we found out that it was illegal. So then, about

six—no, eight months later, we decided we wanted to get married right—before the baby came. Within that time, you know, we had a chance, if we wanted to split we could split, if not, we could end up getting married. So we decided to get married legally.

And I hurt my mother really bad. I made a deal with my husband—this might sound kind of selfish—but I told him, "Well, if we get married in your church, let's baptize the baby in the Catholic church," and he said, "Okay." So that was our deal. We got married in his church, and I felt so bad, because my mom ... nobody in my family—came. Nobody.
They knew about it, didn't they?

Yeah, but nobody came. And his parents were very happy, because—sure, I got married in their church. And my mother was really, really sad, she felt bad, and I thought, "Well, it's my life now. I mean, I have a right to do what I think is right just like anybody else that's married, even though I'm still young." My parents might still like to tell me what to do, but I think like a woman. I think I do, anyways. So I figured, well—I have to be fair, too. I just can't say, "We're going to do this, and we're going to do that." So I was fair with my husband and he was fair with me.

It is a well known fact that youthful marriages do not have a good survival rate, and those who marry while they are minors (under eighteen) have the worst record of all.

In an attempt to reduce the number of early marriages in California, the State Legislature in 1970 passed a bill which sets some special requirements for minors who want to be married. They must have the customary consent of their parents in writing, but in addition, if either one of the couple is under eighteen, they must have permission of the court in order to obtain a marriage license. They are urged to engage in counseling with a qualified counselor, who then evaluates their degree of maturity and readiness for marriage for the benefit of the judge in making his decision. The young man is usually required to show proof of steady employment. The fact that a young woman is pregnant is not considered of itself an acceptable reason for allowing the marriage.

I was interested to learn how the marriage restrictions regarding minors were working in actual practice, and found many girls eager to tell of their experiences in trying to get a marriage license. Two stories have been selected as representative of a great many more.

Eleanor described how she and her boy friend, and her parents and his parents, had tried to get the necessary permission from the court, because, as she said, "You know how parents always want their children to have a nice wedding."

I can remember, we went through all this trouble trying to get married, and nobody would marry us anywhere. The judge had known a lot of young couples, and he was just totally against young people getting married, and he would not consent for anything. We wanted to have a nice small wedding in a church, and we went through counseling sessions with our own minister that I've been with all these years. But we had to have a consent by a judge. We looked everywhere. There were judges that my parents knew, and they thought they could pull some strings, and there was no way. I was sixteen, and Cliff was seventeen. And I was pregnant, and they wouldn't consent to it, you know. Anywhere. We would have to wait until after the baby was born, and we didn't want to do that. So finally—it was a big, long hassle, and I was already three months pregnant—we wanted it all over with and everything, so we went to Las Vegas and got married.

Annette's experience was similar to Eleanor's, but her story contains certain interesting variations.

We had planned on getting married, and we had already saved $400 in the bank before I got pregnant. As soon as I was eighteen we had planned on getting married. So we just went ahead and we got married that summer, because I got pregnant in April.

Did you have a wedding?

Well, we wanted to. We wanted to go to the chapel and invite the family ... but the judge we went to, he let us talk and everything, and right after that he said, "Well, in the first place, I don't think anybody under eighteen, or even eighteen, or maybe even twenty, should be allowed to marry if they are not mature enough to handle it, because there are so many divorces." So he just said, "No."

Then we went to the court in Los Angeles, and they gave us a hassle because you have to have all these papers since I'm under age, and a statement from his work saying that he does have a job, and that he could progress and make more so that he would be able to support a family. They gave us a hassle about that because it wasn't on a letterhead. And that was because they didn't have stationery for their work. It was just a bakery, a small bakery—they didn't have anything.

So we just went to Vegas and got married by court, and came back and had our reception. It was on a Thursday that we went to L.A. and they gave us a hassle at the court and said no. All the invitations were out, and so that night we went to Vegas, and we came back, and he had to be at work on Saturday morning to make our cake, because he's a baker, and he baked our cake.

Although some of the girls were able to meet the requirements of the state law and obtain a license to marry in California, quite a few simply went out of the state—to Nevada, Utah, or Mexico, where regulations were less demanding. Their accounts left me with the impression that the effectiveness of the California law regarding early marriages is open to question; and that although it undoubtedly has reduced the number of early marriages *performed in California*, it has had no real deterrent value if a young couple (or their parents) have sufficient determination and initiative—and the means—to go elsewhere.

CHAPTER SEVEN

Keeping the Child

The fact that every year in the United States nearly a quarter of a million high school girls and junior high school girls have babies and keep them is no longer front page news. It excited consternation and alarm when the news media began to publicize these statistics in the mid-seventies. But for most people now this is just one more problem they would rather not think about — that is, until it turns up in their own family. And when that happens, the private world of that particular family is turned upside down.

If one thing is clear, it is this: someone who is still a child herself, as far as age and legal status are concerned, can not possibly undertake responsibility for the care and nurture of a child of her own *alone*. She requires the ongoing, dependable help of at least one, and often several, adults. She needs expert medical services which she has no money to pay for. She has to have a place to live where a little child will be welcome over a period of years. She needs education, including immediate instruction in child care and child development, nutrition, money management, and a crash course in vocational training.

The realization that she must have help, if she takes on the responsibility of motherhood, often precipitates a drastic overhaul of the total family situation. Frequently a girl's mother feels obliged to give up her own job so that she can care for her grandchild while her daughter goes to school. The young father, very often still in high school himself, will probably have to forego his own educational plans and take a job. In order to make room for one more person in an already overcrowded household, brothers or sisters may have to double up, surrendering some favorite area of privacy. Something has to give. It will not be "business as usual" again until the new young family has progressed to the point of being self sufficient.

This chapter will include an explanation of feelings and thoughts which the girls remembered having as they decided to keep the child. It is well to keep in mind that the word "decide" is not always appropriately used in situations like these, where emotions from within and pressures from without often combine to create a confusing, even frightening state of mind. At times a "decision" is reached because no other possible "decision" can be tolerated. And at times no real "decision" is reached at all, time runs out, and the situation itself becomes in effect the "decision." As the poster so popular in the seventies proclaimed, "Not to decide is to decide."

Some of the girls who were interviewed stated quite clearly that they *wanted to have a child*, but not all of them for the same reason; many had struggled with feelings of ambivalence, and some had rationalized; and there were some who said they did *not* want to have a child, after pregnancy had already occurred. Most of the girls discussed how parents, relatives, friends, or the baby's father advised them. Very few indicated much concern for long-term planning—that is, how they were going to carry out plans for their own and their child's future.

A great many girls spoke of *wanting* the child, even those whose inclination to keep the baby had received its primary impetus from their rejection of any other alternative. It is perfectly normal and natural to love children and to want some of one's own. The following statements leave little room for doubt about the desire for a child.

1 I wanted to have a baby. We had tried and tried for so long to have a baby, and I wouldn't come out pregnant.

2 I've always loved children—and once you finally realize this is happening, and you finally think it through—I knew that I was going to keep this baby, with or without Tom. It made no difference to me—well, I loved Tom, and I wanted Tommy to have a father—but I would have kept him by myself, too, I know I could have managed.

Even when there was no doubt that girls had wanted a child, two nagging questions remained to be answered: Did they want to have a child right then? Had they given much thought to whether or not they were *ready* to have a child? Here are two responses.

1 I don't know. It's funny. I was thinking about it ... when I first got pregnant, I didn't really think of the responsibility, I didn't think of ... the being tied down. All I thought was, "Wow! It's a baby!" And I didn't really think of anything like that. But as the months went by I finally realized it was a big responsibility. And as soon as they are born, you are tied down, and you can't do anything, unless ... you know, you've got a responsibility to yourself and to your kid.

2 I did not know what it was like to have a kid. I had no idea. All I know is, "This is my kid, I'm not going to have an abortion, I don't care what anybody tells me, it's my blood, and I'm going to bear it. God will not curse you with something that you can not handle, that's what my mother has always told me—He will not give you no burden that you can not handle.

Okay ... I did not know that you had to take the baby everywhere you go. I thought you had a definite baby sitter with the grandparents if you're living with them. I thought, you know, all you've got to do is go! ... *No, you don't—no way!*

I knew I had to work—I didn't know this at the time, I thought that—hey, everybody, since I've got a baby, all my friends are going to give me everything I need, my old man's going to give me everything I need ... *Huh-uh, it's not true!*

I didn't know you had to change a baby's diaper every so often, I thought you just had to change them maybe once a day. I didn't know you had to heat bottles, I didn't know babies get sick, I did not know you had to bring them to the doctor for shots, I did not know a baby would wake up in the middle of the night wanting a bottle, I did not know how to hold a baby, I didn't know how to bathe a baby. I was very, very new. I did not know anything.

Sometimes there was a compelling underlying reason why a girl wanted to have a child of her own, as Iris explains. Since infancy she had lived in foster homes, and she and her child were living with a foster mother at the time of the interview.

I found out about my third month, and I told her father right away, and he was excited, too. He really wanted the baby as much as I did. I thought of abortion — it went through my mind for a while — but then I decided not to do it, because I couldn't do it. I talked to my foster mother, you know. I told her what had happened, and she was trying to get me to give her up or have an abortion. I said, "No way." I couldn't do it, you know. A lot of people in the house — they weren't really bugging me — but they'd joke around and say things, you know — "That's going to be a lot of work!" — things like that, but I still didn't want to give her up or have an abortion. I already had made my mind up.

Except for the last part, when we sort of had our doubts. Way back we were thinking of giving it up for adoption. We thought that for about a week and we had already made up our minds, already contacted some adoption agency. And then we talked again, and we just said we'll give it a try. So, we're still trying. I don't think I could give her up, give her away.

In a way I was glad it happened, for some reason, I guess. Because I guess I wanted a family of my own, and she'd be my family.

Sometimes pregnancy was seen as a way to achieve a particular goal — in the following situation, marriage to the boy she loved.

I got the pill for a while. Then I just stopped taking it. I don't know why, you know — I just stopped taking it. I guess I really wasn't afraid of being pregnant, because, you know ... I wasn't afraid of it, like some girls are. Because I just wanted *him*, and I wouldn't mind having his baby, even though I was young. I didn't really think about it very much. I just more or less thought about *him*.

Were you sure that he would marry you if you got pregnant?

Yeah, because we had talked about getting married and we'd go, "Oh, we'll wait a while." We used to talk about it. He used to always say, "Well, I wonder what my kids will be like." I go, "Well, you're going to find out!" And he goes, "Oh!"

The frank statement that follows was made by a girl who was nineteen at the time of the interview. Thinking back to a period in her life three years earlier, she describes the fantasy she experienced during pregnancy. But her remarks lack any expression of joyful anticipation. She stops short of saying she *wanted* the child.

I think I was so young, and I didn't really realize, it didn't faze me. I just thought that I was pregnant, and that I was going to have this baby. I didn't give it, really, any thought. That's just the way I looked at it—like I was pregnant and I was going to have this baby. I didn't think about the consequences or anything, because I didn't know. I had no idea ... Now that I have *her* ... I think about having another one, and I know what it's like, and I hesitate. But then, you know, I didn't know anything.

You think you know what you're expecting and stuff, but you don't. Yes, I knew I was pregnant, but it didn't faze me until she came out and I was in the hospital, and I looked at her, and I said, "Oh, now I have a baby." But the whole while I was pregnant, I kept thinking, "I'm going to have a baby"—but not, you know ... really.

Another girl who viewed her experience from the vantage point of time showed hesitation in evaluating it. More than four years had passed since the birth of her child. Toward the end of our conversation I asked her whether it had been a good thing or not for her to have a child at seventeen. Her reply was a long time in coming, and scarcely audible at first.

No ... But then, she's here now ... But then, it might have been, it was, I think it happened, it happened for a reason ... It *was* for a *reason*. So maybe it's for the best, you know ... like I said, I don't know.

Then there was June, who said she had *not* wanted to become pregnant when she did. During a discussion of birth control, she expressed her feelings.

I never even considered taking the pill. I thought about foam and everything, but I never really got so concerned where I would do anything about it, and I was *stupid*—it was stupid, because I didn't want to get pregnant then. I thought about having a baby and so on, and there were times when I really wanted to, but then I'd come back to my senses and say, "I'm too young, it would tie me down, I'm not mature or anything else." I got pregnant, I was stupid, I should have used something—but what's done is done, and you can't change it.

June's practical approach to a problem situation enabled her to accept her responsibility and do what needed to be done. Not every girl was this calm and self disciplined. Roxanne, for instance, had been tormented by ambivalence early in pregnancy —"I didn't know what to do. I didn't want him, and then I did want him, and I was so mixed up I really didn't know." Then, late in pregnancy, she experienced a surge of negative feelings about having a child that reached dangerous proportions.

We were together until about my sixth month of pregnancy. Then I found out he was seeing somebody else. I got so upset. I wanted to ... I didn't want the baby right then any more. But I was already six months. My teacher told me I was too late to get an abortion. So I just ... for about two or three months I didn't want nothing, you know. And I wanted to ... that same night that I found out, I wanted to jump in front of a car and just ... but *I* didn't want to die ... I was walking beside a wash. I wanted to jump off into that wash, but then again *I* didn't want to die.
This was the night you found out?
Right. That night I found out. I wanted to so much, but I didn't want to hurt *myself*. I just didn't want the baby.

You wanted to bring on a miscarriage?
   Yes. Really fast.

The girls did consult with their parents, but at times the situation was so highly charged with emotion that no rational discussion could take place. Margot described what happened when she was barely fifteen years old.

I knew that first month I was pregnant, and I got scared, but I kept saying to myself that I wanted it. But I didn't know *why* I wanted it. I was scared. I still wanted it, but I was afraid what my mom would say. I told my boy friend—not till three months later—I told him and he said he was happy and everything, but there was nothing he could do because, you see, he's married. So I didn't know what to do then, you know, because he said he couldn't leave her because of other problems they had.

I didn't let my mom know until about the fourth month— actually, I didn't let her know, my cousins let her know. She was real upset, and she just told me that I was going to keep the baby, and she was so upset that she wanted to put my boy friend in jail. And I got upset and said, "Well, I'll get an abortion, if that's what you want." She says, "No, that's not what I want. Now that you got pregnant, you're going to go through with it. If that's what you wanted, that's what you're going to get now."

Then I started thinking when she said that. She started telling me that she wasn't going to help me, I was going to get no help from her, and everything, and that started putting me thinking, "What am I going to do all by myself? He said he couldn't help me." So then I thought—well, maybe I should get an abortion and then tell them I miscarriaged or something. But then I kept putting it off, and then it was too late, so then I went all the way through my pregnancy.

Another fifteen-year-old who consulted her mother received a response that stopped far short of giving her any constructive help.

I thought I was ready to accept the responsibility, and I wanted to go ahead and try—give it my best shot.

What was your family's reaction?

My mom was totally upset about it, and she suggested a lot of things that I could do, like giving the baby up for adoption, turning the baby over to her legally, or getting an abortion when I first told her.

Did you explore any of these possibilities seriously?

I told her, I explained my feelings, and what I wanted to do, and she said, "Okay, it's your life. If you want to ruin it, okay."

In a somewhat different vein, Dora set forth her rationale for keeping her child in spite of strong family disapproval.

The whole time I was pregnant, it seemed like each and every one of them would get me on the side and say, "Are you really happy?" and "Why are you doing this? He's married." Everyone knew he was married. And they would always lecture me. One at a time they did, they'd say, like one aunt told me, "Why do you do this? You have a whole life ahead of you. You could have anything you want, your parents would give you anything you want, because they always have. Why do you want to ruin your life by having a baby?"

And I'd say, "I'm happy. I don't care what happens to me, I'm happy. I have no regrets about having him."

Like one aunt told me, "If you're having it just to get *him*, it's never going to work, because he's already married, and you can't win somebody by doing something like this," and I'd say, "I know, I don't care if I'm by myself. There's other guys in this world, and there's a lot of girls that aren't married that have babies." I go, "Look at him! The girl he married already had a baby from somebody else." I said, "Look at him! He married someone that had a baby, so I can find someone that will marry me. And if I don't, I don't care, I'll be by myself!"

Throughout the interviews, as in the excerpts just cited, I found ample evidence of feelings, of ambivalence, of rationalization—but few signs of any real "coming to grips with reality" during the period when the decision was being made to keep the child—that is, hard-headed thinking based on a girl's own particular situation and the necessity of planning for the child's future. It seemed as though many of them were saying to themselves and everyone else, "Never mind. It *will* work out."

The following excerpt is a rare example of some practical thinking on a personal level at the time of decision making. Ronda could still have gotten an abortion at the time of this incident.

My dad said, "I don't care what you want to do about it—we don't care, your mom don't care." We wrote down pros and cons, to keep it or not to keep it, and they came out *equal!* And then I was doing dishes one day, and he came up and he put his arms around me and he said, "Make me a grand-daddy," and after that I said, "Daddy—well, if I can support it, and I can finish school, I'll do it."

But if I couldn't have done either one, I would have never had it, because I think supporting the baby means a lot, and graduating means a lot, because where would you be without a diploma? I mean—I get a diploma, I can get a job—right? And if I couldn't have done either one, I would have never had him. It was just *my* mind made up.

Although attitudes about keeping the child varied—from enthusiasm, through ambivalence, to a sort of stoic acceptance of responsibility—there was general agreement among the girls about the ways in which motherhood had changed their lives. Two facts were mentioned over and over again: having a child had made them *grow up fast,* and taking on full responsibility for a child had been *hard.* There had been little opportunity for the carefree, happy-go-lucky fun and good times that adolescents normally indulge in, and they missed that. The child's needs had to come first. Those who found caring for the child deeply satisfying in itself—especially if the baby's father was on hand to help—saw this as a challenge, even though it was hard. Those who felt lonely or overburdened were apt to see it as just plain hard.

In the light of what has just been said, why does a young girl keep more than one child if she is unmarried? It's a puzzling question, but the fact that young girls often do keep more than one child was borne out by these interviews. The same resistance to abortion, adoption, and marriage which had influenced decision making during the first pregnancy still prevailed when additional pregnancies occurred. Although three girls who were unmarried did choose abortion for a second or third pregnancy, nine chose to keep the additional child.

In situations where an unmarried couple had been living together for several years, it was easy to understand how a second or third child might be desired by both parents. My chief interest lay in discovering what feelings, what rationale, led a girl to keep more than one child when she could not count on help from the child's father and would therefore have to assume full responsibility for the child herself.

The unmarried girls who had more than one child were very frank in discussing their feelings. Anna Marie, for instance, at seventeen had two babies less than one year apart in age. I asked her how she felt about the close timing.

> Oh, it's not a good idea ... it's *hard!* People say it's easy, but I think it's hard, because when one's sick, they're both sick. And one's crying ... my oldest one wants to be babied a lot, I had to hold him and rock him. The other one's not used to being rocked, because I don't pick him up like I did the first one, as much. It's all right now, but when he was smaller and my oldest one was in a rocking mood, he was just crying, so it was kind of hard, because I couldn't keep up with one and then take care of the other one.

Carol, also seventeen, had given birth to her third child just two weeks before the day of our conversation. I asked her to tell me what her life had been like for the past three years, from the time of her first pregnancy.

> If I had a chance I wouldn't have any—not until I got a little older. It ties you down, it's tiring at times … But I *love* kids, I enjoy them—but I do like to go out, and it's not a picnic, like I said. I like to go out and do things that I can't do, because I have my kids to take care of. When I had one child, it wasn't so bad.
>
> My boyfriend, when we had the first one—it was not like he didn't like kids, he just wasn't into it. Now, he's into it. But at first he wasn't used to it at all, and he was never around no kids, no babies or anything. He didn't ever hold a baby, and now he always holds the new baby. He's kind of used to it now. I think he likes kids now.
>
> My family would tease me and say I was the one that's going to have all the kids. But I'm not going to have any more. I don't want any more. And neither does my boy friend, he doesn't want any more.
>
> I was taking birth control, but the doctor said I might have missed a day. I didn't know I was pregnant the third time until I was six months. It was a shock!
>
> *How did the babies' father react?*
>
> First he said, "Oh no! Not again!" And then he said, "You just *lo-o-ove* kids!" And I said, "Yeah, I love them." Then he just got used to it.

In an attempt to convey some idea of how it feels to be alone with a small child, awaiting the birth of another child, portions of Abbie's story are presented as a conclusion to this chapter. She was twenty when I saw her, living in a small house with her three-year-old child, of whose father she said, "He doesn't come to see us, and I'm glad he doesn't. I don't want anything to do with him." The father of the unborn child had been killed in an accident.

> I didn't want another—like I said, Doug and I weren't getting along. For a while I really wanted one, and then when I

actually found out I was pregnant, it was a while after his death. But just before then I was wondering, "Am I pregnant, or is there something wrong?" I didn't know. I was scared. I didn't want—I was hoping to God that I *wasn't* pregnant. So, yeah, I didn't, you know, *want* another one. I did, but I didn't. I did, but under the right circumstances.

There's a difference between this pregnancy and the last pregnancy. I'm not as brave as I was then. I have a lot of fear. But, of course, I was comforted by having somebody there, and I'm not now. And I know I have to raise two kids by myself.

I feel scared, kind of, pretty *much,* and I feel . . . I don't know . . . I'm not going to reject it, I'm going to love it. Just like my little girl. It's going to be a wanted child. Since I'm pregnant, I'm going to accept it. But to have a better situation—it would be better if I *wasn't* going to have one.

Do you have someone who can care for her for a while, when you find yourself getting too up-tight?

Never—ever, ever! I've been that way many times, where—"God, get me out of this situation! Let me get away for a couple of days, or let somebody take her for a couple of days!" But I've never had that.

Would you consider having another child without marriage?

Well, it really depends on the situation. If I felt totally, totally, totally secure with a man, in every way—I don't mean he has to be rich, but I mean really secure, love-wise—and that I knew wouldn't leave me and stuff . . . it might happen, I don't know.

Is marriage important to you?

I would like to get married, but I really feel it will be a long time before I do, because I want to be really careful. I'm not going to get married if I don't really feel extremely secure.

Well, I think . . . see, if you want to have a child from somebody, whether you're married or not, you're going to have it, if you really want it that bad. And . . . it's hard to explain. Marriage is a lifetime project. I don't want to get divorced, *ever.* If I'm gonna get married, I mean, I'm gonna be really *sure.* If I'm going to have a baby, I want to be really sure, too. I think if I ever have another baby I'd really want to be married. I *think* that way ... but I look at it, and I'm not going to set a standard for myself and say, "I will never have another kid unless I'm married." I can't say that, you know. I'm flexible.

CHAPTER EIGHT

First Sexual Intercourse: Recollections

The first time a girl has sexual intercourse is an experience that is seldom forgotten. Life can never be quite the same again, for the "age of innocence" has ended—even if the age of maturity has not yet begun. One girl probably voiced the attitude of many adolescents when she said, "You're a woman—you really are—the first time you have intercourse you become a woman."

For reasons which elude most adults, large numbers of young people are engaging in sexual activity at ages which a few years ago would have been considered preposterous. One third of the girls I interviewed said they had had intercourse by the age of fourteen; but actually, half of this group that started early had had their first experience of intercourse at age thirteen or earlier.

Since this book is concerned with sexual behavior *only as it relates to pregnancy*, this chapter will be devoted to material provided by the girls on the following topics: the kinds of relationships that led to sexual intercourse by age fourteen or earlier, reactions when pregnancy occurred after a single instance of intercourse, the role played by girls' mothers, and some well remembered accounts of first experiences.

It seemed important to explore the girls' feelings regarding the kinds of situations that had made them want to have sexual intercourse at a very early age.

Sometimes the relationship between a girl and her boy friend had been a continuing one, lasting for a period of months or even years. In these long relationships the prime motivation seemed to be a great need for affection, understanding, acceptance. One girl said she had been having sex for "about a year and a half" before she became pregnant at age fourteen. She commented, "It's hard to explain. I felt like it was because we *cared* enough. I don't know ... I felt that I loved him enough that it was normal."

The relationship described by another girl was of even longer duration, and it too eventually resulted in pregnancy.

> He was just like a guy I could go to for sex. That's all. If I needed any male companionship, I could go to him. It was convenient because he lived right nearby, and we had sex for about six years. About every other day for six years!

Since pregnancy occurred soon after her fifteenth birthday, her active sex life had started when she was nine years old.

A longing for affection was the reason given by the following girl for becoming involved in sex at the age of twelve.

> I did it more or less because I've always wanted to be loved a lot, and my mom was having troubles with my stepdad and I didn't get it from her; my brother hated my guts, I didn't get it from him; and my stepdad was very distant, I didn't get it from him. Me and my mom had lost our closeness a long time ago. The minute somebody opened their arms and said, "Come here! I'll hold you, I'll take care of you, I'll love you, I'll protect you, I'll be your security"—the minute somebody offered something like that, I took it. So that's what happened.
>
> *Did you understand you could get pregnant?*
>
> Yeah. It worried me a lot. Every time, you know, I'd wait for those three weeks to come, or those four weeks, and I'd be on pins and needles—and then everything was all right, everything was fine. I used to worry, I'd say, "No more! No more! That's stupid!" But every time it came right down to it, I just started feeling so warm, and so close, and so loved, that it would completely rush out of my mind.

Several girls brought out the fact that their interest in sex was equal to that of their boy friends, and they had willingly participated in early experiments.

> That was in seventh or eighth grade, and Leo was the first person I really ever did anything with. I wasn't pressured into it— we both wanted to. I knew I could get pregnant, but then I'd

always—you know how you think—"I'm going to be the one not to." Yeah, I wasn't stupid, I knew I could. And the stupid thing was we didn't have protection. But again, I always thought, "Well, I'm going to be the one that doesn't get pregnant." We did use a contraceptive once in a while. He used a rubber a few times—I guess the times we worried about it. And then the other times, you know ...

A girl who "went steady" at an early age talked about how she encouraged the development of a sexual relationship.

I had like a steady boy friend, and he was sixteen and I had just turned thirteen. And he was—I don't know—he's very conservative, and he never pushed me like I'm sure a lot of men would. But he never pushed me, and it was about six months after we had been going out together, so I think it was probably I wanted to, I guess. But he never pressured me.

We went together for about a year. We broke up because he was really busy. He did very well in school and it was his senior year in high school, and the next year he was going to the university, plus he was working, so it just kind of tapered off because he was just too busy. And I demand a lot of attention myself! So it just kind of tapered off.

There were other instances, however, in which the boy was clearly the aggressor, and the girl was reluctant. Anne described how she reacted when she was fourteen.

The first time, the first time I ever had sex, I wasn't with somebody I was deeply in love with. It was with somebody that I had been seeing—just him—for a long time, but I wasn't deeply in love with him ... That was really probably a traumatic thing in my life, because the way I believed, the way I was brought up in, sex is for marriage—which I believe in, you know, *these* days.
So how did you get involved in that early experience?
    Well, I just, I finally ... what it was, was I finally gave in. This guy had been bugging me and bugging me, and finally ... we

had done other stuff before that, I did everything except for going all the way. He was three years older than me ... He was the first one, and then, like I didn't have sex with anybody for maybe a year after that.

Although most often the boys were about the same age as the girls, occasionally a girl became involved at an early age with a man who was much older. Vera, for instance, who admitted she did not really know what sex was all about, became involved at fourteen with a man six years older. Two weeks after they met, she began a sexual relationship with him.

This was my first. He told me that if I was ever to get pregnant, that he'd take care of me. And he'd want the baby ... He used to drink, and he used to take reds a lot. And, like I was mostly scared of him, because he would take pills, and like when we were going together when I was pregnant he would like threaten to kill me, and he would hit me and stuff like that ... He started going out with somebody else and he didn't want to see me no more, so we just broke up. And I just had the baby, and he never seen the baby. He's never seen it.

More than one girl mentioned alcohol as an important factor in her first experience with sex. Amy still seemed a bit mystified by what had happened to her four years earlier.

It was really strange ... well, see, the point was, is, I really didn't want to do it. But guys have a way of getting you involved in it, like getting you drunk. And that is what happened to me. I got drunk, to the point where—hell, I didn't know what was going on.

If a girl fully understood the nature of intercourse, she was aware that pregnancy could result. The following case, in which the girl was fourteen and the boy was a year younger, raises— and answers—a totally different question.

Well, I never thought I would get pregnant, but I knew I *could*, you know ... But I didn't know if *he* was old enough to, you know, *get* me pregnant ... Yeah ... But it seems he was!

Although most girls acknowledged the part their own interest and desire had played in their introduction to sex, for at least a few the first episode had been a shocking experience which had occurred when they were twelve or thirteen years old. Only one of these girls was able to give a coherent account of what had happened.

I was only in seventh grade, and the boy was twenty-eight years old, and he'd take me for walks. I didn't know what was happening. I wasn't even old enough to really know what was going to happen. I thought he was trying to hurt me, you know. That's what I thought—he was just trying to hurt me. And he kept telling me he loved me and stuff ... I had a real bad experience. And I was really scared.

I was really afraid of—every boy is going to do this, it's going to hurt me, they're going to hurt me—so I was really afraid. I was really afraid of boys. I was afraid that if they kissed me they were going to hurt me, and every time a boy tried to kiss me, I'd cry, because I'd think ... it was a bad experience.

Quite a few girls had run away from home—some repeatedly. And sometimes the first experience in sex took place in a strange locale with strange people, under circumstances that left much to be desired.

I met him when we were at a snack bar when I ran away from home, and I didn't have no place to go. My shoes were falling apart. I was living with this girl, and all she wanted to do every day was go off here and there. She had a house, but she never stayed home. She'd come home maybe four o'clock in the morning and leave around eight o'clock. She was just hyperactive.

I had a fever and I was sweating and I was throwing up, and she was telling me, "Come on!" So I'd be down at the Boulevard—I'd be down there till two o'clock in the morning—and

I'd be sick and I'd be sweating and stuff, and I didn't have no shoes or nothing, I'd be coughing, and I'd go into a friend's apartment to lay down all the time. And I got tired.

I met this guy, and he told me I could come and live at his house. And I was just so happy to have somewhere, you know — shelter. So I was just happy. And me and him, we fell in love. We really loved each other, and he wanted to marry me. I asked my parents and my parents said, "No."

My probation officer wanted me to straighten out, so he sent me away for a while, and when I came back I was still in love with him. But he had changed. He had started taking heroin, started using drugs. I found out he was going to bed with other girls and going out on me. But I loved him so much I used to forgive him all the time. And it just went on like that and finally I just broke up with him.

Although the length of time sexual intercourse had been going on before pregnancy occurred was not routinely discussed in all interviews, it was specifically mentioned by 77 girls, with over half (44) reporting that pregnancy had occurred within six months. Some added that it must have happened on one of the first few occasions, or "right away practically," as one girl remarked.

Especially significant, however, is the fact that six girls became pregnant as the result of *a single instance* of sexual intercourse — their very *first*. They could pinpoint the occasion precisely, because there had been a considerable lapse of time before they had had intercourse again, if ever.

No matter how old or how young the girl was, the most common reaction when pregnancy resulted from a single instance of sex was shock.

Well, I wanted to experience it myself, I had heard things, you know, but I didn't think — wow! — *once!* — why would I get pregnant?

And it took place sometimes under the most unexpected circumstances.

We were fighting over my hat—he had taken it from me. I have a lot of hats— I like hats. And he had taken it from me, and we were arguing over that, and wrestling and stuff. And then it just kind of happened.

Like so many others, the girl just quoted had brushed aside any consideration of the fact she could become pregnant, believing that to be utterly impossible. "I blocked it out of my mind," she said. "I figured this was my first time and I couldn't get pregnant."

The fact that there was only one instance of sex seemed to intensify the feelings of remorse and guilt which the previous training of certain girls would have generated anyway. Two made special reference to this.

Nicole was only fourteen, and had been brought up in a strict religious family.

I don't know if I said this before, but we only got in trouble just once. And we were both sorry after, that we had gotten in trouble and everything. Because you know, we ... I don't believe in doing stuff like that with just everybody. I mean I always said—like if any other guy ever tried to get me like that, I just told him, "Hey, when I get married I don't want to tell my husband" ... well, you know, whatever ...

Although Charleen was nearly three years older than Nicole, she also felt a sense of guilt because she had ignored the teachings of her church.

One night it just happened. That was the first and last time— just this once. I felt kind of ... it wasn't a peace inside of me, you know, until I got it right. It's mostly having to do with church and stuff. They tell you that's wrong, and you're not supposed to do that, that's the wrong way to be.

It is curious, and also ironic, that although most girls could count on their mothers to help them care for a child once it was born, rarely had these same mothers been able to provide their daughters with basic information, and a chance to discuss their anxieties about matters of sex, *before* they became pregnant.

Take Maureen, for instance. She had been sexually involved with Bill for a long time — three years, in fact — before she became pregnant.

> I was thirteen, I think. Me and Bill, we went out a couple of times and had a real good time, and we just talked a lot, and you know, we just got closer and closer. Gradually, we just started talking about it one night, and after about a week of talking about it, just decided that we'd do it.
>
> *Were you concerned about getting pregnant?*
>
> Well, I was never told the facts of life, ever — I was never told about it, so I didn't ... see, I thought — this is stupid! — see, I thought that you could not get pregnant unless you were married. That's just how I thought. I think things would have been different if I was told what could happen if you do this. And you know, I was never told anything.
>
> *Did you ever ask your mother?*
>
> Yeah, a couple of times. And she just said, "Oh, we'll worry about that when you're older. It's not important."

Even when a mother had conscientiously tried to give her daughter essential information about sex at a reasonable age, the emotions and the tension that the girl felt as she became involved in a sexual relationship created a barrier between them that neither one could overcome.

> I knew all the facts about sex when I was in the eighth grade. My mother told me.
>
> *Did you feel you could talk to her about it?*
>
> No, I was embarrassed. She would tell us about it, but it wasn't like — me and my mom were close, but we weren't close enough to where she would come in and ask me what my problems were and I'd tell her. So I'd usually tell my best friend. I can't keep problems to myself — I just can't — it would bother me too much. But it was just embarrassing to ask my mom. I didn't want to ask her. She would be one-sided, and like, "No, you can't have those feelings, you're just too

young." And if you have feelings, you're going to have them. You can't control them. The emotions are there—they over-power you.

I am convinced that most parents would like to be able to help their children through difficult periods in their lives. But very often, by the time the children have a critical need for help, their parents are unable even to *reach* them, let alone communicate with them. Sometimes the over-riding desire to spare a son or daughter the hardship and the heartache they themselves have known turns them into nagging, ineffectual guardians that can only warn or threaten, without explanation.

Paula, who became pregnant at sixteen in spite of warnings and restrictions, tells how her mother went about trying to protect her.

> When I'd go out on a date, I'd have to be in by eleven. On the day of my formal, I had to be in at midnight. All my friends could stay out till one or two, and I used to tell my mom, "You're holding me down too much." Then before I'd go out she would say, "Don't get pregnant!" and this was even before we started to know each other really good. And I'd tell her, "I won't."
>
> Yet if I'd go somewhere she wouldn't trust me, she'd have one of my brothers or sisters go with me. Like my little sister—she ended up going to Magic Mountain with us, and I mean, what could you do over there? Just have a good time! So here I'd have a little tag-along sister, in the sixth grade! I thought this was too much, and I'd tell my mom, "You know, even if I have a little chaperon around, I still could do things that you don't know about." Then she got really upset, and she wouldn't let me go out for a long time.

Occasionally there was a notable exception to the general rule that communication regarding sexual matters between child and parent is difficult, if not impossible. Lucy felt comfortable with her mother, and asked her for advice when she was thinking about having intercourse with her boy friend.

We were talking about marriage, and my parents really liked him. And I don't know, I always thought ... well, I'm not going to do that until I'm married, it's just not right.

And then, I really cared a lot about him—I cared a really super lot. And I talked to my mom, I discussed it with her before I did anything. I said, "I really love him a lot, and I want to share something with him that I've never shared with anybody." And she said, "That's okay. If you want to do that, there's nothing wrong with that. If you love somebody, there's nothing wrong with it. But if you're just doing it to be doing it, don't do that. Do it if you feel in your heart you're right." About a month later we did it.

For most girls, the occasion on which they first experience sexual intercourse is indelibly impressed on their minds. One girl told me, "I was fourteen years old," and then proceeded to cite the exact date *four and one half years earlier,* when she had first had sex. This is not to say that it is unimportant to boys, but the nature of a boy's experience is very different from that of a girl. Both know for the first time the physical closeness of the merging of two bodies. But the girl's body *is different* after her sex life begins. She has let go of something which up to that time she had held onto—her virginity. To be sure, boys speak of their "loss of virginity," too. But it is not the same.

Nadine was in ninth grade, going with a high school senior. They had grown very fond of each other, and both wanted to explore sex. She was curious, but she was also afraid. I asked whether she thought it would be an enjoyable experience.

Well, the first time I tried it, it wasn't! ... It was a good two months before we actually made it, because—like we tried it three times before and it hurt too bad with me, so we stopped. When we finally did break through, you know, I passed out on him, and I woke up in a puddle of blood. The only thing I can remember is him standing there, scared to death—'cause he was all bloody, I was all bloody—and he was just standing there. I looked at him and I said, "I'm never going to do this again!"

Then I guess it was just the relation I had with him that cured it, because he didn't leave my side that night at all. I laid on the sofa because I hurt terrible, and he just stayed there, and he just laid there and patted my hand or held my hand, he was touching me constantly the whole night, and it just made us so much closer. I was the first he ever had, to take the cherry from, he was my first I'd ever done anything with.

Although boys are more apt to be aggressors when it comes to early sexual experimenting, sometimes girls take the initiative. According to Marion, what motivated her was a sort of scientific curiosity.

I was really and truly interested in reproduction itself, I guess I was always interested in it from the clinical point of view. People can't understand it, but I really was. I knew about the male and I knew about the female, and I was wondering—how in the heck does it work? Well, I was going to find out for myself, and I did! And I enjoyed it.

Pressure from friends to engage in sex has long been associated with the adolescent male. Today, however, peer pressure is frequently a compelling factor in the case of young girls. Lillian at fourteen, for example, had felt pressured by her girl friends to discover for herself what they all had been describing as something new and wonderful.

Paul and I had been going out for about seven months, and all the time everybody was saying to me, "Oh, you can't be a virgin still!" And here I was—I think back, I was just fourteen years old, I was practically a baby—and everybody was saying, "Oh, it's the greatest, and you'll love it!" and everything. And I was curious, I'm a very curious person. So I thought, "Well, I've got to try it."

Paul and I had talked about it and he said, "No, no, I'm going to keep you pure," and everything. So it was quite a while after the first time we talked about it that we did anything. But I was drunk. I was drinking lemonade and vodka. At four o'clock in the afternoon, I said, "Well, come on in the house," and I was already bombed. And so—I was sitting on the kitchen counter, and I said, "Aw, come on," you know, "it's not going to kill you or anything!" and I was putting him down like, "Are you afraid? I bet you're a virgin!" and stuff like that. So he said, "Okay."

He took a drink, and we went in my bedroom, and I can tell you exactly what each of us were wearing, and the way my room was arranged, and everything. And it wasn't all it was cracked up to be. I mean, you have to get used to it, but I didn't expect, you know … it was *painful!*

Some teen-age girls really do not understand what is involved in the act of sexual intercourse. Peggy did not, at age fifteen. Her mother had tried to explain it all to her when she was nine or ten, but her explanation had been confusing, and Peggy had failed to understand it. What she did know was that she did not want to lose her boy friend.

We went to the drive-ins for about seven months every Friday and Saturday night, and I fought him off. Through the second movie he pouted and was mad—well, not actually mad, but he didn't understand. He thought I didn't want *him.* I didn't know really what it was all about.

Then the one night I got disgusted—I just said, "Forget it!" In the back of my mind I thought that if I gave in, he'd get it and I'd probably never see him again, and I was afraid to lose him, but it seemed like I wasn't keeping him. I didn't want to keep him just for him to come down on weekends and make love and stuff, and I didn't want to lose him for giving it to him either. I didn't really know what I wanted.

So I said, "Forget it!" and we did it. I was so afraid. I didn't know what he was going to do, and what it was going to be like, or anything. I was totally scared to death. For me it was not a great experience.

The story which concludes this chapter illustrates a type of exploitation which is often practiced on teen-age girls who have just begun to "date." It was told by a girl who had described her childhood as rather hectic, with little opportunity for enjoyment of the good times most children take for granted. For instance, she had never been to Disneyland. When a young man asked her to go there with him, she accepted eagerly.

The guy took me to Disneyland for dinner, and went out to the beach afterward and said, "Okay, pay me back." And I said, "Take me home." And he says, "No." I thought, "What am I going to do? Have to do something, I've got to get back home. I'm 'way out here at the beach with a kook." ... So, it *hurt* ... but I got back home, and I never saw *him* again. I told him, "I *never* want to see you again!"

See, I didn't really know what to expect. I didn't know the whole thing involved. I had been to sex education, but I never knew it was that traumatic. I didn't know you had to go through guys saying, "Aw, come on!" ... I had never been through that. It was done in a car, and I didn't want to do anything in a car. I didn't know it could be done in a car. He was older than I was, and stronger, and I didn't want to fight. So, I just said, "Take what you want, and leave the rest. Leave me alone. I want to go home."

That night, that one time when I was sixteen, when I went to Disneyland, that was my first time to ever be there. And he took me to dinner, and then he took me on the Cup and Saucer, and then—we left. And I so much wanted to stay there, and just *play!*—go every place!—and ... nope!

CHAPTER NINE

Attitudes toward Birth Control

Since most teen-age pregnancies are unplanned, this raises a puzzling question. Now that contraceptives are available, why does any girl become pregnant unless she wants to?

This deceptively simple question is so important that most of this chapter will be devoted to an attempt to provide some answers to it. For until this question is thought through, there will be very little progress toward an understanding of birth *control.*

According to available evidence, fewer than ten per cent of pregnancies among unmarried teen-agers are intended, and the experiences described by the girls I interviewed would seem to bear out that statement. The great majority expressed surprise, shock, and even disbelief when they discovered they were pregnant.

With few exceptions, all the girls were aware that sexual intercourse could lead to pregnancy. So I asked them if they had *worried* about becoming pregnant. Here are two replies.

1 Yeah, we did talk about it, you know. I worried about it, but — it seems like you know it, but you don't. I don't know ... it's so *dumb,* when you really think about it, because we didn't ever plan on doing it ... it just happened, you know ... Well, *afterwards* I was worried.

2 Just took a chance — and we blew it! I guess it was our own fault, and we know it *now,* but we never really thought much about it before.

Now those girls knew that there were such things as contraceptives, but a great many young girls have been kept completely in the dark about this whole subject. Francine, for example, who became pregnant when she was fifteen, put it this way: "You know, you don't hear too many people talk about birth control until you get pregnant."

When I asked another girl if she thought it would have helped her and her boy friend if they had had more information before they became involved in sex, she made the following comment.

> Yeah, probably about birth control. We never heard of it. It's funny. I think that in schools—the high schools and probably the junior highs—they should have something about birth control—sex education—but they don't.
>
> The high school here, they do have a sex education class, but it's not until you're about a sophomore, and girls are getting pregnant out of the seventh grade. That's too late!

Jean took the need for birth control information a step further with this observation.

> They should teach you *that* in school. In sex education, they tell you how to get pregnant, they don't tell you how to *prevent* it.
>
> My mom told me how to get pregnant, too, just like the school did, but not how to stop, you know.

Knowing that contraceptives exist is only a start. Teen-agers have to know much more than that if they are to be able to use them. For instance, they have to know how to *obtain* contraceptives. Belinda explained her state of mind when she was fourteen and having sex.

> I always knew there was something to take for not getting pregnant, but I didn't know where to get it, and then again, with my mother finding out ... Because if I would have known, I would have taken it. I know now how easy it is to get it. And if I would have known that, I would have gotten it.

Then there is also that common human frailty, procrastination, to be reckoned with. Even when a girl knows there is such a thing as birth control, and also knows where she can get it, she often puts off doing anything about it.

I always thought I should take something, but I never really—I just kept saying, "Well, maybe tomorrow." Tomorrow never came. I was in a rush, I thought maybe something could happen, but yet, when you're so in love, you don't think like that. You don't think, "Well, it could happen to me," or anything like that.

The role that fear plays is very important. There is first of all the understandable fear of becoming pregnant when one is not ready to have a child, but there are other fears in a young girl's mind which sometimes actually outweigh the fear of pregnancy. Louise described her fear of the pill—an attitude shared by many of the girls.

See, I was afraid to take the pill because of the things I had heard about the pill—sometimes you can get cancer and stuff—which my doctor said isn't really true. And I just wouldn't take anything. I was afraid to take birth control, but I just took the chance of getting pregnant.

While the fear of possible dangers inherent in the pill is a specific fear, which can be dealt with in a logical manner by seeking advice from a doctor, there are other anxieties that are more emotional in nature than rational. For example, the fear of parental disapproval of their behavior keeps many girls from discussing birth control with their mothers.

Telling your mom that you need birth control, because of something ... you know ... they get kind of shocked and everything. I didn't want to ... I'd rather ... you know ...

And then there is the feeling often described as "fear," which is really embarrassment. Many girls mentioned their embarrassment, or fear, about going to a clinic to request contraceptives. Claire, however, was specific.

Do you know why I didn't want to take birth control? Because I didn't want them to examine me—that's why. That's the only thing that really stopped me. Because I didn't want a pelvic exam.

Since few, if any, of the girls had very much knowledge of the facts of reproduction, they were apt to "put two and two together" in what seemed to them a logical sequence, and then draw their own conclusions. Several allowed themselves to be lulled into complacency regarding the risk of pregnancy because they had concluded that either they or their boy friends were sterile, as two of the girls explained.

1 I said, "I think I better get on the pill." And weeks went on and months went on, and I still hadn't got on them. And we were having sex and I still didn't get pregnant, so I thought, "Well, maybe I just can't get pregnant." And he said, "Well, maybe you can't." So I just didn't go down there and even get them, and I think it was a month later I got pregnant.

I just didn't think I could get pregnant, so I didn't have any reason to go down there. Because I thought once you had sex you get pregnant right away.

2 We didn't really think we were going to have a child, because Shane thought for a while that he was sterile ... until I became pregnant. And he's not sterile!
What made him think he was sterile?
Well, he'd done it with this other girl, and she had never gotten pregnant, and nobody else he had ever had had gotten pregnant, and so ...

When I asked the girls if they had ever really talked about birth control with their boy friends, I found their replies varied widely. There were those who frankly admitted that there had been no discussion at all.

I don't know ... now that you say, you know ... it's kind of funny how we didn't even think about it, you know. We never said nothing about that.

Others tried to get some discussion going, but didn't get very far with their boy friends. Like Billie.

Yeah, it worried me—really it did. But he says, "Don't worry about it." He kept on saying, "Don't worry about it, don't worry about it." Then when I did wind up pregnant he said it was my fault.

And there were a few girls who saw no need for birth control under the circumstances, with everything looking so rosy.

We was going to get married, you know, and we was going to be happy-go-lucky. He told me, "If you get pregnant, bear my child, and I'll marry you." And we *was* going to get married — but *I'm* the one that didn't want to get married.

This tendency to attribute special value, special significance, to everything her boy friend says and does is a common characteristic of adolescent girls. His promises, his desires, his beliefs, his likes and dislikes — all are apt to be acceptable to her. She has often cut herself off from her parents during this period, and therefore willingly casts her lot with him, and him alone.

I was worried, but he was the type that don't worry. And that's what he'd tell me, "Don't worry. We'll get you checked if you are. Don't worry about it." And if I was, he was going to help me get an abortion. I didn't like it or anything, but I felt it would probably be the best thing.

He was even thinking of getting me the pill from work. He would say something and I would get my hopes up, and then he'd never do it. There were days that I went to school crying, I'd say, "Art! Art!" and he'd just say, "Don't worry about it. Don't worry about it."

Did you never think of getting birth control on your own or with your parents' help?

With me and Art's relationship, my parents were totally out of it. They loved Art dearly, but when it came down to me and Art, just nothing was said. My relationship with Art, and Art's relationship with me, was kept totally out of it.

I don't think he intended on getting me pregnant. It was one of those things that just happened. I would ask him, "Art, we've got to go down. We've got to go down!" And he would just give me all kinds of love and hold me, and I'd cry and everything, "Art, what'll I do? What if I'm pregnant?" And he'd say, "Don't worry about it." And just the way he did it—he's got these big brown cow eyes, you know, beautiful brown eyes, and you just look at them and you just believe everything he says. And you just kind of melt and think, "Okay, everything will be all right. If he says it's going to be all right, it's going to be all right."

But not all of the girls had set their men on pedestals. Some had pretty bitter things to say about what they perceived as refusal on the part of the male to take any responsibility for birth control. Here are two comments.

1 They don't care. They say they love you and everything but they still don't care. They know that nothing is going to happen to them. No, the girl gets pregnant ... let her take the responsibility. It's her fault. She wanted the fun and games.

2 A lot of the guys won't use condoms. That's the only thing—most of the guys won't. "I ain't going to use those things!" They carry on like they're a bunch of idiots, and they won't use them, and that's usually why the girl goes on the pill—'cause the guys just ain't going to do it. Whether you like it or not, they're just not going to.

After reflecting on her own experience, and then generalizing from that, Edith had arrived at a no-nonsense conclusion.

He never brought up the subject of birth control. I did. And I have a feeling for some reason that when they bring it up, they feel like they have to be responsible for it. If they bring up the subject, then they better be ready to take the responsibility to use a condom. And I have a feeling that most men for some reason shy away from that idea, and until they come up with something more attractive to men, that men are always going to shine the responsibility onto the women.

In the emotional turmoil in which they found themselves, were any of the girls able to confide in their mothers and ask them for help? It was not to be expected, in view of the uneasy relationship most adolescents have with their parents, that many would have felt they could tell their mothers they wanted information on birth control. But their replies to the question were by no means all alike.

Some girls did not even try to find out whether their mothers would discuss birth control with them. They simply *assumed* they would not.

> It's good if you have a mother that understands, but if you have a mother who, when you ask her something, right away her voice starts to get a little bit higher than usual, you're afraid to ask, so you just don't talk about it.

As Beryl looked back on her experience, she realized her mother would have been willing to get birth control for her, if only she herself could have admitted freely what she wanted to do—before it was too late to do anything.

> She would have been upset, but she would have handled it. She would have gotten the pills for me. I was just too scared, I didn't want to hurt her, you know.
>
> When I was already pregnant but I wasn't positive, she told me that if I was doing something, that she'd help me, she wanted me to get on the pill. Not to get pregnant and mess things up. I was too young right now and had school and everything. But I kept telling her that I wasn't doing anything. I felt pretty sure that I was already pregnant, and I wanted to tell her then, but I was just too scared.

Avis, on the other hand, at seventeen had obtained birth control pills on her own and was taking them. She described her mother's reaction when she found out about the pills.

> When she found my pills, she said, "You're not supposed to be taking these! You're not even—what are you taking these for?" And I didn't want to tell her, you know. I just said, "Because I wanted to take them so they would regulate my period."
>
> She emptied them all out. Then she said, "You're not supposed to be on these things. If you're doing anything—you're

not supposed to be doing anything! Who do you think you are?" That's all she told me ... Just like when I got pregnant, she goes, "Who gave you permission to do that kind of stuff? You're not supposed to be doing that kind of stuff!" and I didn't say nothing.

After Avis had had her baby, however, her mother's viewpoint changed.

When I went for my six-weeks check-up, she said, "What are you going to take?" And I was surprised that came out of her — her that threw my pills away, her that wanted me never to do anything! I said, "I don't know." She said, "You got to take something, you just can't be without anything. You never know." She told me what she thought I should do, and she explained everything to me.

The remarks made by the following girl resemble some that have been previously quoted. This girl and her mother had never discussed contraceptives and she felt very anxious about having sex without any, but she never seemed able to get to the clinic on her own. Then she got pregnant. As she talked about her mother, I sensed that their relationship was basically a good one, and so I asked her what she thought her mother might have said if she had been able to come right out and tell her mother she was having sex and wanted to get some pills.

I think she would have *let* me. I think she would have taken me to the doctor's and let me gotten on. Because we talk about all this stuff now — but we never did before. So I didn't know. I was scared. I didn't want to say anything to her because I thought maybe she'd give me a big lecture.

But no matter what they say, you're still going to do it, you know. And I know she would have rather me gotten on pills because she *knows* there's no way she can stop me from having sex.

The difficulties which many teen-agers face when they try to obtain contraceptives on their own are enough to discourage all but the most determined and the most resourceful. Even if they know *where* to go, they may not be able to get there at the right hour because of school. They may need transportation, which usually means persuading a friend to take them. And they are not always sure they are doing the right thing. In other words, if they muster the courage to go, and have everything finally arranged for, they have usually exhausted their supply of stamina and can not handle any further complication.

My sister took me to some place down in L.A.—one of those free clinics, you know. We stayed there for about six hours, and the doctor I had there was really putting me down for being there, you know, and he sort of started scaring me: "Do you know you could die?" and this and that, and this and that—just got to scare you. Then he goes, "Do you have a gynecologist?" and I go, "What's that?" And he goes, "Well, if you're going to be doing this kind of thing, you should know ... " your vocabulary, and all this kind of stuff. I just didn't say anything—it wasn't worth the hassle. So I got the pills ...

Then my sister started talking to me, "Are you sure you want to start taking them?" and started telling me all the side effects, after I got them. And then I decided I didn't want to take them, because I was afraid of certain things, and I wanted to go back and get a diaphragm. But my sister said, "I'm not going to help you any more. If you want to do it, you've just got to do it on your own."

The doctor described in the preceding story was obviously not comfortable discussing birth control when his patient was an immature teen-ager. In reality, there are quite a few doctors who prefer to avoid the topic of contraception if it involves young girls. The following episode occurred when sixteen-year-old Kate and her mother went together to consult a doctor.

Right before I got pregnant we went to the doctor's. She wanted me to get the pill, you know, just in case, 'cause she knew I was going with him for a long time. My mom just asked the doctor, when I had my physical, if maybe he could give me the pill because I was going with somebody, and he said, "She's too young. You shouldn't let her take those, that's just pushing her," and all that stuff. And my mom said, "No, she told me she'd like to take them."

He told my mom, "Well, she doesn't need them. She hasn't done nothing yet." And I *had* done something—that's why I don't understand ... And my mom says, "Well, she's out messing around and I want her to take them. I'd rather have her taking the pill than be pregnant."

So he said, "All right. I'll just write a prescription and I'll send it to you. It'll be in the mail," or something. And finally, when we got it, it was too late. I was pregnant, so I didn't have time to take them.

Later on in our conversation, Kate told me she wanted to wait several years before having another child, and was taking pills and having no problems. I asked if she had gotten the pills from the same doctor she and her mother had consulted.

No, this is a different doctor, a gynecologist. And he makes sure every time I walk in that door, he says, "Are you taking your pills?" And I say, "Yes."

He made me take them from the first—well, right after the baby was born he sent them home with me, and he told me, "As soon as you stop bleeding and I see you after six weeks, then I want you to start taking them." He didn't want to see me coming in, getting pregnant again, you know. So he was really nice.

The girls were more than willing to discuss the experiences they had had with various forms of birth control. Though relatively few had been seriously practicing birth control prior to the birth of their first child, most had become interested in limiting the size of their families and spacing any additional children.

Their stories were full of accounts of trial and error. All the standard methods of contraception had been tried by one or more girls, or their husbands or boy friends: the rhythm method, withdrawal, foam or vaginal suppositories, condoms, the pill, the intra-uterine device (IUD), the diaphragm, and even sterilization (vasectomy or tubal ligation). And *every single method except vasectomy* had, in one or more instances, failed to prevent a pregnancy.

Why?

It is one thing to think of birth control in the abstract, and quite another thing to add the human factor; yet it is essential to take into consideration a person's life style, home situation, degree of maturity, and emotional stability when discussing birth control.

My conversations with the young mothers revealed that during the period before the first pregnancy the high level of motivation so necessary for success with birth control was most often lacking. Many were afraid of it, or felt guilty or embarrassed about asking for it. They didn't always follow directions carefully. Some knew nothing at all about birth control.

Since all the girls, however, had received medical care at the time of childbirth, most discussed some type of contraceptive with a physician when they went for their six-weeks check-up. It was then that they usually gave up relying on do-it-yourself methods (withdrawal, condoms, rhythm, or foam), and decided in favor of the birth control methods that require medical supervision. For the majority pills were prescribed.

It is easy to assume that all should go well if a girl uses a contraceptive method prescribed by a doctor. But for a great many of the girls there were serious problems even then.

Problems with pills were generally of two types: those which were caused by failure on the girl's part to take the pills according to directions, and those involving physical suffering caused by the side effects of the pills.

The first kind of problem is illustrated by the following frank statements which help explain why many teen-agers do not succeed with pills.

1 See, I had been taking birth control pills before then. But then I said, "Why should I taken them for and I ain't doing nothing?"

Then, the time I stopped taking them I started *doing* something. So *that's* what happened!

2 I didn't like it because, you know, you have to take them the same time every day, and I was in school, and doing different things. I was never home, and I never carried a purse so I never had nothing to keep them in—so I just got all mixed up with that, you know. I'd never be taking them all the time and everything. So—I just forgot about them.

There were those who followed directions correctly, but suffered unpleasant side effects—nausea, weight gain, or, as in the following example, excessive vaginal bleeding.

I'm always having my period, practically, except about one week of the month. It's a drag. The doctor says it's the kind of pill, because—you know—a certain amount of estrogen, or something like that. I've tried two kinds of pills. It gets to be irritating.

There were some pregnancies reported by those who were taking pills—pregnancies which they felt were not caused by failure to follow instructions, but by failure of the pills themselves.

The following story was told by a girl who had obtained pills, with her mother's approval, soon after she had begun a sexual relationship with her boy friend.

I went back to the clinic because I was spotting blood really bad. So I asked them for stronger pills, because I knew that was the problem—they weren't strong enough. And they wouldn't give them to me. They told me I'd have to wait until my first year was up, until I had another Pap smear, and then they'd give me the stronger pills *if* I really needed them. But I told them that I had been spotting blood really bad and everything, and they said, "Well, keep on taking the ones you've got until your year is up." I had another month to go before my year was up.

So it ended up I got pregnant on the pill, and I never skipped a day or nothing.

Side effects with the IUD included bleeding and cramps, which often subsided after the initial period had passed. But there were instances of more serious trouble—for example, when the IUD became lodged in the wrong place. In the following story, an IUD which had been inserted when the girl first became sexually active failed to prevent a pregnancy.

When I first found out that I was pregnant, I rebelled. "It couldn't happen to me! I'm the only one it happens to!"—you know, the whole bit. And then, I had had the IUD inserted, a special shield which is the only thing a girl can get single, if she hasn't had a child before. They said it was 98 per cent safe.

When I found out I was pregnant, they took it out and said, "You're pregnant." The nurse goes, "You're one out of the two in a hundred that ever get pregnant on this." And I go, "Terrific! Where's the other one?"

They told me I could lose the baby. When they pulled the shield out, I started bleeding, the whole bit, and they told me most likely I had lost the baby. I was kind of glad, kind of sad— I was mixed a million. So they took another blood test—it was there—and I go, "Terrific!"

In spite of all the problems associated with birth control, most of the girls said that they were practicing birth control, in one form or another, at the time they were interviewed.

It is interesting to note that a few had decided to utilize the very oldest form of birth control—*abstinence*. They were simply going to avoid having sex—at least for the time being. Two unmarried girls expressed their viewpoints on this.

1 I've had a couple of chances with boys I like since I had the baby, and I still say "No," because the fear of having to go through the pain and suffering again is the best birth control for me.

2 It's not that I don't really like it, but it's … to me it's really

important, it's an expression of love, and before I will have sex with someone I'm going to love him, or care for him a great deal … and be sure that they're not going to leave me hurt, you know, really bad … that they do care about me.

The others were using conventional types of contraceptives, under doctors' direction. Some were experiencing no problems whatsoever, others had tried several methods before finding one that was tolerable, and still others were coping with unresolved problems. But they were persevering for a purpose, which was perhaps expressed most accurately in the following statement.

I do use pills, birth control pills. I really don't like having to take them every day, you know, but I don't like the idea of being pregnant every year, you know.

CHAPTER TEN

The Birth Experience

Doctors regard teen-age pregnancies as "high risk." This judgment is based on the findings of medical research which show that girls in their teens are much more likely to have serious problems during pregnancy and childbirth than are women who are just a few years older.

Some of these problems, like prolonged labor, occur mainly because teen-agers are adolescents—still growing. Since their pelvic bone structure is not yet fully developed, a baby's head is sometimes just too large for normal passage through the birth canal.

Two diseases associated with pregnancy—toxemia and anemia—occur far too often among teen-agers. Both are serious and require prompt medical attention, but both can usually be avoided altogether if a prospective mother has good prenatal care and proper nutrition.

A third area of concern involves the babies born to very young mothers. These infants are much more likely to have low birth weight (under five and one half pounds), even when they are full-term, than the babies born to women in their early twenties.

These are some of the reasons why doctors have labeled teen-age pregnancies "high risk." The trouble is that teen-agers do not *know* the special risks they run if they become pregnant, because no one has told them. A great many girls, as a matter of fact, do not even know what the signs of pregnancy are, and they are much too frightened to find out. So they prefer to ignore worrisome symptoms, and hide important changes that are taking place in their bodies, and this combination of ignorance and fear constitutes one of the prime reasons why teen-agers have so many problems during pregnancy and childbirth: *inadequate prenatal care*. They frequently put off seeing a doctor till very late in pregnancy, when serious problems may have already developed. Worst of all, the very youngest girls—those at highest risk—are the most likely to be avoiding everybody, including doctors. The ironic truth is this: *the younger a girl is when she becomes pregnant, the less likely she is to receive prenatal medical care.*

The accuracy of this observation was reinforced by the young mothers I talked with. The only ones who had received absolutely *no prenatal care* were four who were between twelve and fifteen years of age when their babies were born. All of them had concealed their pregnancy from their families—and to a degree from themselves as well—until time of delivery. All four recounted stories of their childbirth experience in vivid detail, but only one described what had happened during the long, lonely period of pregnancy.

This was Rosalie, who at fourteen had relegated any notion of pregnancy to some obscure corner of her mind. Even though she began to experience problems brought on by her pregnancy, she just kept diagnosing herself, or relying on the advice of a friend of her mother's who was a nurse.

Pretty soon the baby started kicking and that's when I started to worry. I could feel the weight that was kind of like a bowling ball. So I consulted our nurse friend, and she said, "You probably have a bowel blockage," and I said, "Whatever that is." And she said, "It feels kinda heavy inside, kind of like in your intestines," and I could feel it, and I thought that was probably what it was.

After a while, Rosalie's legs and arms became badly swollen—"just ballooned up big"—but her mother was inclined to attribute most of her complaints to hypochondria. "My mom quit believing me a long time ago," she said. Finally, when abdominal pains began to occur frequently, her mother took her to a doctor.

I told the doctor about the pains I was having Tuesday night and that day. He pushed on my stomach, and he asked me all kinds of questions, and then he said, "All right, go ahead and get dressed."

When my mom went into the office, he told her, "I'm ninety per cent positive her spleen is enlarged, and her liver is enlarged ten times what it should be. Her stomach is big, but it has a kind of hardness to it that the rest of her body doesn't." He said, "I think she has leukemia."

This doctor had her mother take Rosalie to a hospital for further examination. Tests for leukemia had already started when one of the physicians said, "Let me check her out — we've only got one diagnosis." Very soon he began to suspect pregnancy, though Rosalie stoutly maintained that was impossible. The x-rays which the doctor ordered revealed the skeleton of a baby in her abdominal area. But the doctors could not detect a heartbeat.

They told me the baby was dead, but inside I felt him moving around, and I thought, you know, "He's not dead." But I didn't know what kind of condition he was in — I'd been eating nothing but junk food, and with the emotional problems I had, I drank a lot, the hard stuff — vodka, tequila. Any time I wanted it, all I'd have to do is call up my friends, "Hey, come over here and party." I thought, "I don't know what kind of condition the baby is in, I don't even know if he's going to have all his arms or his legs. But I know he's alive."

Rosalie went into labor a few hours after the examination. The baby that was born that night did survive, and he did have "all his arms and legs," but both mother and child nearly died from toxemia. "Our hearts kind of gave up," said Rosalie.

Although the most extreme cases of lack of prenatal care were found among the youngest girls, fear and panic often gripped many of the older girls as well and immobilized them during the early period of pregnancy. They did not usually consult a doctor until after they had told their parents about the pregnancy, and frequently months went by while they were figuring how to do that.

One seventeen-year-old girl simply could not bring herself to tell her mother, and more than eight months had gone by before a "busybody" finally got hold of her mother and divulged her secret. Then it was the mother's turn to panic, and it was not until the doctor had demonstrated her daughter's condition to her on the examining table that she could begin to accept the reality of the situation.

> So the doctor came in and I laid down like that, flat on my back, and you could see that I was pregnant. And my mom was asking the doctor, was there any way that I could get an abortion. And he goes, "Oh no! You see, from here to here," he was showing my mom, he goes, "this is a *baby*. This is a *full-term baby!*"

Even after a girl's initial fears had subsided and she was receiving care and advice from a doctor, she was often in emotional turmoil still because of *anxiety*—worry about the future, and especially about the attitude of the baby's father. In my conversations with the girls, I was impressed by the fact that if the boy friend was happy about the pregnancy, and wanted to get married, for example, a girl's whole outlook brightened. She could relax a little. She could focus her attention on decisions that had to be made and tasks that had to be undertaken. She was no longer facing the unknown alone. She could at last concentrate on preparing for childbirth, and on following her doctor's instructions.

If, on the other hand, the baby's father had abandoned her, or if his own doubts and feelings of insecurity only increased her own anxiety, a girl was likely to suffer from a variety of physical complaints and to be negligent about following medical advice. In other words, certain physical complications seemed to have been induced, or intensified, by a girl's emotional state during pregnancy. Gwen, for instance, told how an emotional shock had precipitated a bad attack of asthma, which in turn endangered her unborn child.

> Well, I'm an asthmatic, and when I was six months pregnant, that's when I found out that her father was father of another

child at the same time, and the child's mother was at that time a very good friend of mine. And I was wondering why all of a sudden my friend had stopped coming around, my good friend, and it was very upsetting. And I just wanted to know. I figured, "Well, he doesn't really care too much about me," but I wanted to know if he actually could do a thing like that.

I did call him, and I asked him, "Is this true?" And he said, "Of course it's true." And it really upset me, and I had a very bad attack, and I guess they thought I was really going to lose the baby, because I was hospitalized for about four or five days, and after that I just determined, if there's any way I could, I'm going to have this child, and it's going to be healthy, and I'm going to raise it the best way I can.

Quite a few girls had been bothered by excessive gain in weight, which they attributed to compulsive overeating. Two girls, for instance, said they gained fifty pounds during pregnancy. "After being a size five, it's just awful to think of yourself as a size sixteen," remarked one of them. The other was more blunt: "Well, I sat around and ate like a damn pig. Seven months spread!" Overeating is usually triggered by emotional problems, and the following story illustrates how an unhappy living situation contributed to a weight problem during pregnancy.

All through my pregnancy I couldn't take it at my mom's house, because she thought I was her slave. If I didn't get everything done, she'd bitch my head off. I stayed there for a while ... and I stayed with Hal and his parents for a while. But I couldn't take it there for long either. For a lot of reasons, I felt like I was an intruder and I was living off of them. They were feeding me and stuff, but ... I was just idle ... there was nothing for me to do. Sometimes I'd say to Hal, "Please take me for a walk. Just walk around the block with me. I don't want to turn into a blimp." I ended up weighing 205 pounds before I had the baby, because they ate really fattening things.

Gabrielle's emotional state during pregnancy was characterized by actual resentment about being pregnant, and she engaged in some bizarre behavior that endangered her unborn child.

> I didn't want the baby. I'd try to hit myself in the stomach and everything so I would have a miscarriage, you know. And I'd take a lot of pills—all kinds of aspirins, all kinds of pills of my mother's and dad's, pills that he had gotten from the hospital and stuff. I'd take all of them. I'd take a bunch, and I'd just get sick and I would throw up. And I would just say, "Why can't I die?" And sometimes I'd run fast, and I'd trip and I'd try to fall, and stuff like that—so I wouldn't have this kid.

Fourteen girls mentioned having had miscarriages, either before or after the birth of the child they kept, while they were still of school age. In five instances, the miscarriage had occurred when the girls were only fourteen or fifteen, and the families of these girls had no idea they were pregnant. In fact, some of them never did tell their parents about the early miscarriage, but managed to get medical treatment with the help of a relative or friends.

Two who were fifteen when the miscarriage occurred gave contrasting accounts of the experience. The first girl had seen no reason to modify her life style just because she was pregnant.

> I thought that I wanted a baby, you know. I'd seen some of my friends that are older—about seventeen years old—and they had babies, and I kind of envied them, and then when I got pregnant, I thought—you know—"I won't be able to have a baby."
>
> I used to sniff paint—while I was pregnant, too—and I was at a park and they had some big high thing, and I was loaded, and I fell off of it, right on my stomach, and I was about—almost four months. I hit my stomach real hard, I hit every part of it. I started laughing after I fell, you know, and I got up, and I said, "I'm all right." My friends all panicked, because they knew that I was pregnant. They picked me up, and were telling me all kinds of stuff for falling down.
>
> When I got home, I started bleeding and it scared me

because I didn't know what was wrong. I never experienced anything like that, so it scared me, and I started getting like pains in my back, it was hurting me. My mother didn't know I was pregnant, and I didn't know if I should go and ask her for help or something. I got up finally, and I asked her for help, because I didn't know what to do, and then afterwards she took me to a hospital, and they gave me a D and C.

The second girl, who had her heart set on having a child, became so despondent after the miscarriage that she attempted suicide.

I had a miscarriage when I was almost two months pregnant. I really wanted that child.

I bled and bled and bled, and it scared me to heck. And the doctor, who I really didn't care for that much, was very rough. Since I had to go back after I lost it, and he didn't even know that I'd lost it, I showed him the "thing," I kept the "thing." He says, "Oh no, it's nothing." So when I went back about two weeks later and had another pregnancy test (I was still bleeding at the time), it came back negative. And I knew that I lost the baby the day I lost it. There was still that glimmer of hope, but I knew better.

Emotionally, I cracked up. I tried to kill myself. I was taking drugs constantly, because I couldn't face what had really happened. So one day I just said, "I can't take this any more." My best friend gave me a bunch of pills—her parents had a bowl just brimming with different kinds of pills, all prescribed. So she said, "Well, take your pick." So I took twenty-four pills.

The relationship between the girls and their doctors was not always one of mutual understanding and respect. After all, both were faced by an unusual situation. A doctor generally expects anyone under eighteen to be accompanied by a parent, and consequently he may feel a little uneasy when he has to deal with a fifteen-year-old on a one-to-one basis. On the other hand, an adolescent girl is usually unfamiliar with medical procedures, and may appear resistant and difficult when she is actually only scared. Unfortunately, unless the doctor makes a real effort to understand the girl's feelings and win her trust, she may become resentful, and ignore medical advice.

The girls had a good deal to say about their doctors, but their most common complaint was that the doctors didn't take time enough to talk with them.

> The doctor had so many patients that he'd take you in the room and check you over, and kind of like throw you out. He wouldn't ask you if you had any questions, he wouldn't take time to explain anything.

Occasionally they got the feeling the doctors were "putting them down."

> I'd go for a check-up, and they'd just check me out and walk out. Oh, they'd say one thing to me, "You're getting too fat," or "You're gaining too much weight. You need to go on a diet." They gave me a slip one time that said, "Diet Food," you know, but they weren't encouraging at all. They were negative. They walked in with a straight face, checked the baby's heartbeat, and walked right out. They never talked to me, they never let me ask them any questions, and when I did, they'd answer as briefly as possible and that's it.

One of the girls, who had obtained prenatal care at a clinic in a large hospital, made some astute observations about the quality of care she had received.

> I thought they were regular doctors, and I found out after I'd been going there for a few weeks they were interns. And I wanted a regular doctor, I didn't want an intern. But it was too late. I had already been going there a couple of months—so I just stayed there.
>
> The rooms are right next door to each other. They're just like stalls. You could hear the girls in the other rooms asking questions, and the interns told every girl the same answer to their questions. Like if I'd say my back was hurting really bad,

he'd say, "Oh well, that's just the pressure of the baby." And every time someone else would tell them that, they'd give them the same answer. Then if something else came up that they weren't sure about, they'd go out the door and go down the hall and ask the doctor, and the doctor would tell them what he figured it was, and then they'd come back and tell you. And that's what I didn't like—they weren't absolutely sure.

He told me the baby was already in position, all ready to come out and everything, her head was already down there—and I ended up having a Caesarian because she *wasn't* in position like they said she was.

But there were also doctors for whom the girls had nothing but the highest praise. All of these doctors had been willing to take plenty of time to put their young patients at ease, and to explain things to them. Marina made special mention of her doctor's willingness to wait out the long hours with her in order to let her give birth to her child naturally, if possible. She had had to change doctors late in pregnancy. The baby was long overdue and very large—"too big for me, since I'm only five feet and I shouldn't have a big baby."

This doctor, he's a really good doctor, and he cares about his patients. Like some doctors will figure, "Well, I don't want to be here for seventeen hours. I'll just give her a Caesarian and get it over with." This doctor—he's a really good doctor—he took his time, he called every half hour, and was really concerned about me. And he said, if I needed a Caesarian, he would give it to me, but he was going to wait. He was really good.

As time for delivery approached, the way a girl felt about it depended a great deal on whether or not she had had adequate instruction and preparation for childbirth. Some girls attended sessions where particular methods were taught, and others depended on the instruction provided through the special classes for pregnant girls in the schools. Husbands usually took instruction with the girls and acted as coaches, and sometimes unmarried fathers also took the classes. If the father of the baby declined to assist, a girl's mother often volunteered to take the training and stay with her through labor and delivery.

My husband and I had six weeks of classes. When the time came, we acted like we had had ten kids or something. It was about twelve midnight and I started laboring, and he just went back to sleep. I told him, "I think we'd better go," and I called the doctor. We went to the gas station, put gas in the tank, and we just went up there real calm, and we went through the labor and delivery. Everything was really calm.

He cut the umbilical cord, he bathed the baby, and he was real calm about everything. He enjoyed it, he was really happy!

One of the girls described the birth of her daughter as a positively exhilarating experience, both for her and for her husband, and gave the doctor credit for making it so.

This doctor's philosophy is that pregnant women aren't sick, and that the husband and wife are there at the time of conception and they both should be there at the time of birth. See, the doctor delivered the head and the shoulders, and my husband delivered the rest of the body — which was fantastic! He got a kick out of that!

It was not just a coincidence that those who were the most anxious, afraid, or depressed, were apt to be those who had had no instruction at all, and so were totally unprepared for childbirth. Two sixteen-year-old girls made the following comments.

1 I didn't know anything. The only thing — my mom told me that the pain was so bad you could die of a heart attack. She really got me scared. When I started labor I didn't know what was going on.

2 Well, people told me, you know, how it hurts ... and some people say it don't hurt ... it depends. And I figured it was just an experience that I'd have to figure out myself. But when it

happened, it hurted ... the pains ... and I didn't think it was going to be like that.

Had you had any classes to prepare you for childbirth?

No, because the baby's father was put away, and my sister, she had to go to school, she has classes at night, the same night that they had La Maze, and nobody else would want to go with me. So I didn't go. I just signed up for it.

Even when ample instruction had been provided, in addition to good medical care, the casualness of the teen-age life style often prevailed at critical moments.

I was at the swap meet at the time when the pains started. All day since they started, they weren't five minutes apart, and they just annoyed me—they didn't hurt. We were selling stuff there that day.

We came home about four o'clock. My mom got all nervous, and she called the hospital and asked them what we should do, and they said to bring me in. *Then* I got scared.

In school they taught us, when you start labor, if you eat anything you'll get sick, and I never got sick, and I was eating all day long. And on the way to the hospital I was eating a corn dog, and I didn't get sick. So I wasn't sure, again, if that's what it was. When I really got scared was when they checked me and everything, and then they went out and told my mom and my boy friend that they were going to keep me.

Planning for every possible eventuality as delivery time approaches does not come easily to most adolescents. Arranging for transportation to the hospital at the right time, for example, can be a big problem. In Kit's case, delay in reaching the hospital resulted in painful tearing which might otherwise have been avoided.

Well, I got to the hospital at eleven-thirty, and he was born at twelve-forty. I was really fast. When I got there, they said they could see the crowning of his head already, because ... see, I had to wait so long at my stepsister's house. She had to get dressed and everything, and while I was waiting for her the baby was just coming.

See, all morning long I was in labor, and I was just sitting there, I didn't want to say anything because I was scared, and I just kept getting up and down. And all of a sudden I just started bleeding a lot, so then I finally told her.

The doctor told me that if I would have come earlier, then he would have given me a saddle block. But it came so fast. Afterwards he gave it to me so I could rest, because it took about three hours to sew me. And it took about a month and a half to heal up.

Although most of the girls had hoped to be able to experience natural childbirth, and many had tried to prepare themselves for it by attending classes and practicing the proper techniques, in nine cases the babies (including a pair of twins) were delivered by Caesarian section.

Bernice, who seemed to have the best understanding of just what had happened, and *why* she had to have the surgery, gave this account.

After he was a month late, I was going to get my bag of waters broke. And that morning when I was supposed to go in, at five o'clock my water broke, and I went in, and I was in labor for about twelve hours. It was pretty hard labor, and they took x-rays. The doctor had told me the night before that it was possible that I'd have to have a Caesarian. So about five o'clock that night they took me in the delivery room and I had a Caesarian, because he was too big. He was really big—he weighed nine, six and a half!

I didn't have enough room. If it had been a normal size baby … His head was almost fourteen inches around, so there was no room for him to pass through.

Several girls told of having Caesarian sections because the baby was in breech position. In Heidi's case, there were complicating factors. She prefaced her story with the remark, "It was scary" and, under the circumstances, that seemed an understatement, considering the long, anxious wait she endured while doctors decided how to deal with her problem.

I went in at eight o'clock on Sunday night, and they checked me and said that the baby was feet down, and one leg was turned behind her back, and the cord was wrapped around her neck. And then my water broke, and the foot started through the birth canal. But because the other leg was turned, she wouldn't ... there wasn't enough pressure, and they said even if I did, that it was possible her leg could be broken and she could get strangled. They took me in for x-rays about ten o'clock that night. They didn't do the Caesarian until two o'clock the next afternoon.
Why the long delay?
Well, they were hoping maybe they could turn her, you know — get her back up and turn her — and that didn't work. I was in a clinic where I had interns and residents, and they ... let's see, how did it work? ... One of them checked me, and he couldn't give the okay for a section. So they had to call in another doctor for an opinion. So, they got the other doctor's opinion, and then they had to call in the chief-of-staff and get his okay, and after that happened, they couldn't find the anesthesiologist. So by the time they got everybody in, it was two o'clock on Monday when she was born.

Although most of the babies born to the girls who were interviewed were sound and healthy, there were also some who had gotten off to a rough start in life. Eleven weighed less than five and one half pounds at birth. All except one of these infants survived. Several, however, required intensive care in the hospital for weeks. The two smallest, one weighing only two pounds and the other weighing three pounds, four ounces, remained hospitalized for eight and six weeks respectively.

The baby that died was the second child of a very young girl. Hannah's first baby, born when she had just turned fifteen, had weighed less than six pounds at birth. When this child was three or four months old, Hannah became pregnant again. She went to her doctor, and told her young boy friend, but did not discuss this second pregnancy with her mother or others in her family. "I never told them until after I lost her," she said.

That must have been a very hard thing for you to go through.
Yeah, it was.

Had you thought, when it happened, that you might terminate that pregnancy—have an abortion?
Yeah, I wanted to have an abortion, but my doctor didn't believe in it. He said at my age it would be really hard for me and that it might kill me.

At what point in the pregnancy were you talking to him about it? Was it very early?
It was early—it was about my third month. I said, "Well, I can't keep it, it'll be too much for me." And he said, "You can do it, you can do it." He doesn't give abortions, he doesn't believe in them at all.

The baby was born prematurely, at seven months, and lived only one day. When that happened, Hannah was not yet sixteen.

Besides the babies that had low birth weight, a few others had health problems during the early days of their lives. Of these, breathing difficulties and jaundice were mentioned most often. All the problems had been corrected, or were being treated, however, and they were described in great detail. The deep concern which these young mothers showed for any child who was sick was unmistakable.

It is impossible for me to say with certainty what effects the stress and anxiety which characterized the lives of so many of the girls during pregnancy may have had on their childbirth experiences and on the condition of their babies at birth. One of the girls, however, made some interesting comments along this line which are suggestive, when she compared and contrasted her own experiences with her two children. The first, Kelly, had been born when she was seventeen, and the second, Chrissie, when she was twenty.

With Kelly I was in labor for twenty-four hours, back labor the whole time. My husband and I went to the La Maze method together, and if we hadn't hung onto each other there would have been nobody to hang onto. My parents resented me. They cared and they helped, but it was painful for them, too.

This last delivery was incredible. It was so easy—I couldn't believe it! I had a very good doctor, and I delivered her myself—from the shoulders out. I reached down and delivered her—and walked out of the delivery room! It was fantastic, and I could tell you six hours about it! It was great!

It was really beautiful. They put her right onto my chest and I massaged her back, and after they cut the cord they wrapped her in a blanket. My husband was there, and he held her immediately following. He was so happy! It was nice to see his face, because when he was in the delivery room with Kelly, he was petrified. He was just too young. He wanted to, but he wasn't ready for it.

Chrissie is totally different from Kelly. The difference between the two kids—I'm sure it has something to do with their personalities—but Kelly never did sleep through the night, never, and Chrissie was sleeping through the night at maybe a week old ... And I tried to nurse Kelly—I know a lot of this is attributed to my age, the age difference, and the experience— but I tried to nurse Kelly and she became allergic to my milk, so I had to take her off. Chrissie I nursed until she was almost six months old, and she's been very docile, very peaceful, and so much stronger from the beginning.

The difference in the two—I can't attribute it totally to personality. Because they are sisters. I think a lot of anxiety during my pregnancy with Kelly contributed to it.

CHAPTER ELEVEN

Attitudes toward School

We are accustomed to thinking of the schools as second only to the family in the amount of influence they exert over children's lives. Five days a week, most children spend more of their waking hours in school than at home. Legally, they have no option but to do this. While families may require their children to do certain things—like attending church, doing chores, or being home by nine o'clock—it is the State that requires children to attend school.

During recent years, however, the authority of the schools in the matter of attendance has become seriously eroded. Though in former times the threat of the truant officer was enough to drive any wavering student through the school house door, today the schools are finding compulsory methods ineffective. Because of continual changes in school population within a given district, even keeping accurate records of attendance becomes a problem. Families often move without notifying school officials. Unless they register their children in the new district, school authorities there have no way of knowing that these children exist. Also, if both parents of a child are away from home all day at work—an increasingly common situation—it is difficult for school personnel to reach either parent to discuss a child's lack of attendance.

The general public in days gone by adopted a rather complacent attitude about school attendance, simply assuming that all children of school age went to school. Now, however, the situation in some school districts has reached the point where it would be more accurate to say that students are going to school *if they want to go.* And a great many, both boys and girls, are dropping out of school altogether, as early as the ninth grade.

Through my experience with young mothers as a social worker I came to realize how difficult it is for a girl to return to school after the birth of her child. Accordingly, I had accepted without question the statement that, in the country as a whole, the principal reason why girls drop out of school is pregnancy.

Now, however, my conversations with the young mothers have made me question the accuracy of that statement. Although quite a few of the girls had dropped out before finishing high school, in a number of instances they had dropped out *before* they became pregnant. And ironically, some of these same girls had eventually returned to school *because* they were pregnant.

Before students actually drop out of school there is usually a long period of "ditching"—skipping classes, or whole days and even weeks of school. This is the way one girl described her attitude toward school in eleventh grade.

> I used to ditch a lot. They said that I could do real good in school, but I just didn't care about school at the time. I just didn't like it, and so I wouldn't go. I'd be with my boy friend or just be with some girl friends—just wouldn't go to school, that would be all.

Barbie began to ditch in the ninth grade. I asked her where she went when she wasn't in school.

> I would go to the store and get myself some cottage cheese and go play cards. I had a girl friend, and we would always go play cards together on somebody's lawn. We'd only ditch about four classes and we'd play cards all that time, and lunch. Then we'd go back to school. And the next day we'd ditch a couple of these classes, and take lunch.

Another girl explained to me how easy it was to "work the system."

> I wasn't in trouble, but I should have been. I was always one step ahead of being caught. In my sophomore year of high school I think I went only three days. So all the other times I was off fooling around somewhere.
> *Didn't the school get in touch with your family?*
> No, they never called to check on me. They never did

anything. I had a girl friend write all my notes for me.
Where did you go when you didn't go to school?
   Oh, to a friend's house, the beach, the mountains ...

I asked the girls what action the schools took when a long absence occurred, and their answers amounted to, "Little or nothing." Rebecca began to wish they *would* do something.

For about a month I never went to school, and I always expected letters at home. I used to stay at this friend's house. I used to go over there every day, and I was so scared that the school was going to come and see my mom, or that something was going to happen.
   I wanted to go back to school after that. I had missed school for about a month, and I *wanted* to go back. And I said, "Well, maybe I could go back and tell them I was gone on vacation ... but they'll ask my mom, and I don't know what she's going to do." But I didn't know how to get myself back into school — so I stayed away from school. For about three months I didn't go to school. I never got no letters, my mom and my grandmother never got no phone calls, nobody ever came out to the home. I never went near the school, and they never showed up. That made me feel like they didn't care — so I shouldn't care. So I never went to school for about three months.
   Well, they finally did send somebody to the home, and that's when my mom found out. She said why haven't I went, and I said it was beginning to be so long I didn't know how to get back into school — so I just stayed away from school. After I went back, they put me on like four hours a day, and I couldn't do that either. So I stopped going ... I would go, but like only once or twice a week.

In contrast to the stormy reaction truancy would have caused among parents of an earlier generation, the parents of very few of the girls I talked with made much effort to improve their daughters' school attendance. One of the girls, who had been ditching frequently and driving other students around in her car, did report that she and her mother were called into consultation by school authorities, and as a result she began to take school seriously again. Generally speaking, however, parents seemed unmoved by school reports of excessive absence. Dee revealed how she felt about this.

They'd send your report card home, and it says how many days you're absent.
And did that shock your parents?
Yeah, it really did. Because I would leave in the morning when I was supposed to, then I'd go to a friend's house, and I'd come home about the time I usually came home from school.
Did they make a big fuss when that report card came home — all those absences?
They'd look at it, they'd say something for a few minutes, and I'd say, "Yeah, sure," and I'd walk out. That was about it.
Are you really saying that you wish your parents had shown more concern ... ?
Yeah, I wanted more put down, I wanted a foot to put down.
Because ... what would that mean to you if they had?
More love. More security.

Of course, no system that demands compliance with certain requirements will work unless those who are affected by them are willing to *accept* discipline. People can make a mockery of any set of rules — if they want to. But the stories just presented, of Rebecca and Dee, have other elements in them which suggest a longing for more direction and guidance in what was for them a confusing world. Janelle takes their train of thought a step further.

I've always been undisciplined. My mom was always undisciplined. I don't mean getting in trouble — I mean undisciplined about myself, about keeping my house clean. I'm a lot better now. I was very undisciplined for a long time about organization and stuff — organization of my life and of my school work. I mean — if I really would have planned things out, everything could have been different. If I really would have got involved in ... you know, I would have needed someone to help me get organized in my thoughts and my plans ... but if I would have done that, my life would have been a lot more successful.

Do you think kids need to be helped to set goals for themselves?

Sure! And they need to be taught how to organize their thoughts and their plans. I remember in school they talked about goals a lot—"What's your goal for this and that?"... but that didn't help me at all, you know. I mean, really *organize* your thoughts and your plans.

Of course, helping students plan how to reach certain goals requires a great deal of individual attention. And that was the point made time after time during the interviews: the girls said they wanted teachers to be interested in them as persons, and to meet their individual needs. A girl who had dropped out of school in the eleventh grade commented, "I think if there had been a teacher that would have kind of coached me, even a *tiny bit*, it would have helped me."

Polly had a contemptuous attitude toward most of her teachers: "The teachers go, and they sit, and they hand you papers and they say, 'Do it.' And that's it. It's not really an education. You're going because you're being made to go, and they're teaching because they're getting paid for it." But in discussing the teachers she had had over a four-year period, she paid a rare tribute to two.

In fifth grade, the teacher—I liked her. She taught me how to read. I didn't really know how to read, and I didn't really like to read. And she got me to where I liked to read and I knew how to read.

In sixth grade I had a teacher, and all he would do was talk about the Navy. He was in the Navy, and that was all he would talk about.

I enjoyed the eighth grade (I hated seventh grade!). I liked the eighth grade because I had a really good teacher. And if you had problems, you could go talk to him. Nothing was forced on you. You worked at your own speed, and you more or less did your own thing. You had to get your work done—but you were able to do it at your own speed and at your own pace and everything. And I really enjoyed that.

He'd sit down ... there were four classes and four teachers, and we'd get all four classes and four teachers into one room, and sit around in a big circle. He'd start a discussion, and everybody would take turns saying what they thought about it—one person at a time. You know how, when you get a group together, everybody jumps in—right? Well, the whole purpose of his class was self control, self discipline, and courtesy for others. In the classes the key word was "chaos." If somebody said the word "chaos," you sat still, you didn't say a word, you were quiet. It was just automatic. And I don't know ... it was really good. That's the only time I enjoyed school after the seventh grade.

The desire to "go at your own pace," which Polly mentioned, was expressed by a number of girls. Those who needed to go more slowly than the average student argued for this approach, but so did the quick learner who longed to forge ahead. The prevalence of this feeling partly explains why many of the girls preferred continuation schools to regular high schools. Although in certain areas continuation school is still used as a "dumping place" for unruly students by school administrators, it is gradually acquiring a respectable identity of its own. Renee told an amusing tale of her efforts to escape from the traditional system.

I was totally dissatisfied with the regular public school system. They were on a trimester system, and they issued you a work-sheet: "This is what we're going to do this trimester." I had gone from September to October. I was finished, and I said, "Okay—now what should I do?" And they said, "Well, you sit here until next trimester." And I said, "Well, can't I get credit for this, and go on and do something else?"

I knew the continuation school, and I knew that you could work at your own pace there. So I thought, "Gee! If I could find some way to get kicked out of school so I could go to continuation school, then I could work at my own pace, and then I'd be happy." But I couldn't find a way. I tried cutting school, I did everything I could think of. They wouldn't kick me out of school, and they kept saying, "You're such a good student, we're going to give you another chance." And I kept saying, "But I don't *want* another chance. Kick me out! Throw me out! Let me *do* something!" But they didn't do it.

When I got pregnant I said, "Okay, I'm pregnant. Now you have to get rid of me." But they said, "Oh no! You can stay here for a while if you like."

It is ironic that Renee's pregnancy at a very early age proved to be the justification for her eventual transfer to continuation high school. On her own she discovered that there was a special class for pregnant girls, and it happened to be located in the continuation school. She enrolled at once, made rapid progress with her academic requirements, and received her high school diploma at the age of sixteen, when her child was five months old.

Although no other girl chose to play the activist as persistently as Renee, several complained, as she had, that the schools failed to challenge them. It is possible, of course, that they were not trying very hard to accomplish anything, and preferred to sit back and criticize instead; but for whatever reason, the schools held no interest for them. They were just marking time. One girl put it this way: "I didn't feel I was learning anything in the classes. It was just like a big baby sitting thing."

I kept wondering, however, whether teachers and counselors had tried very hard to find out *why* there was so much dissatisfaction on the part of certain students, for I learned through talking with these girls that often underneath their apathy, or outright rebellion, were emotional problems which so absorbed their thoughts, and drained their energies, that studying and attending classes lost their meaning. Anna's story illustrates this point.

I started messing up in school when I was in about the ninth grade.

Now what do you mean by "messing up"?

The wrong crowd, cutting school.

What made you do this?

I don't know. I was shy in seventh grade, and in eighth grade I guess I was just tired of being a "no one," and I decided I was going to do something to get attention. And I started messing around.

Did you have problems at home?

Oh, my mother and me didn't get along. I started running away.

Had you never gotten along, even when you were a little girl?

Well, when they got a divorce, I blamed it all on her. And then we just had conflicts ever since then.

How old were you when your parents were divorced?

Five.

And were you very much aware of what was happening?

Well, I knew that ... I knew what divorce was. I didn't understand why, but I knew what it was and I didn't like it. At that time, I blamed it all on my mother. She left him, and she messed the whole thing up. It probably would have been the opposite if I had been with my father. But I had to blame somebody and take it out on somebody.

When you started to skip school, what did the school do?

Detention. Staying after school—that was all.

Did they talk to your mother?

Oh yeah! She tried really to stop me. She'd restrict me at home. And that just made it worse for me. Because I rebelled.

What kind of things did your crowd do? What did you do for fun?

Hang out somewhere and drink.

How were you feeling about yourself then?

When I was out, I was happy. When I was with the crowd, I was happy. When I got home and started thinking about it, I felt bad for my mother. I didn't want to hurt her. And I didn't know what I wanted.

While rebellious students like Anna, who "mess around," usually come to the attention of school authorities sooner or later, some of the quiet, withdrawn students, who never cause "trouble," may be masking serious depression. Two girls provided prime illustrations of this. The first, only fifteen when I saw her, had expressed her thoughts throughout the interview with unusual clarity, and made use of an extensive vocabulary. I remarked that she must get very good grades in school.

No. Ever since about the middle of the seventh grade, I gave up on school. I had a lot of emotional problems, and I just didn't want to hassle with school. I'd sit through class, and I'd either sleep, or relax, or talk.
Why don't you like school?
I love school! My IQ is 140. I love school, because I love to learn. But it just wasn't important to me after all the things I had to hassle through with my mom and my life and everything. I lost interest in school and learning—because I was so down on life and I was so down on what I'd seen. It wasn't worth it to me. If I would have died the next day, it wouldn't have mattered a bit to me.

The second girl, aged seventeen, said she had begun to skip school before she became pregnant, but the problems created by her pregnancy deepened the sense of depression she already felt. I asked her what she did when she didn't go to school.

I went down to my friend's house—she's an older woman—and talked to her. Because I felt so depressed sometimes. I just wanted to be alone. And then, when I found out I was pregnant, I went down to her house, too, because I needed someone to talk to. Because the situation, you know … John didn't want me … and so I had to talk to somebody. I just couldn't go to school and sit there in class and cry.

From talking with these young mothers I got the distinct impression that they felt traditional high schools paid very little attention to students with personal problems, and that there was no one on the staff they could turn to when they needed help. This was especially evident when the girls were discussing the anxious weeks they lived through after they realized they were pregnant. I asked if they had talked their problem over with anyone at school. Here are two replies.

1 At our school — well, at most schools, I guess — everyone hates the dean, and there was no one there you could go and talk to. We had counselors, but they didn't really listen. They'd say, "Uh-huh," and so on, but that was it.
What about teachers?
It was just their personalities. I never felt I could really confide in them. I didn't feel close enough to them.

2 I almost did go, a couple of times, to one of the English teachers. I'd get up the nerve to tell her, but then I'd think, "No, what if she goes and tells everybody?" Because there were a lot of teachers in school like that.

As I listened to the following story, it became apparent that several adults at Lavonne's school had recognized her plight, but did not want to risk an offer of help. Instead they looked the other way. She was seventeen, attending regular high school, and in her ninth month of pregnancy. The fear that had taken possession of her had made it impossible for her to tell her mother. Yet deep down ...

Did you tell anybody at school, like the school nurse or a counselor?
No. I didn't tell nobody.
That must have been a very lonely, difficult time for you.
It was. I was so scared.
Did anybody at school notice that you were pregnant?
No ... well, just after they found out I was pregnant, some people said, "I thought you were, but I didn't say anything." Some of my teachers — my P.E. teachers especially — said, "I knew something was wrong."
But nobody took you aside and said, "Can I help you? Maybe you have something on your mind?"
No, I wouldn't like that. I would have started crying.
But would it have helped to break the ice? — to tell your mother earlier?
I guess so.

Because your mother had to know some time.

Yeah. I know. That's what I kept saying to myself, too ... I think it probably would have helped—if somebody would have.

In California some schools allow pregnant girls to remain in the regular high school program. Others refer them to a special class designed to meet their needs, where they can stay until the end of the term during which they give birth. But school policy regarding pregnant girls is not always thoroughly understood by all teachers and staff members, or publicized among students, and accordingly many girls, like Lavonne, go unnoticed and unaided.

Shyness, embarrassment about changes in their appearance, and the lethargy or weariness that frequently accompanies early pregnancy are problems that are well known to all those who try to persuade pregnant girls to continue in school. Without assistance and encouragement from understanding adults, many choose the easy way out—staying at home.

I didn't feel like getting up and going to school every morning. I was lazy then. When I was first pregnant, I was real lazy, and I just didn't feel like going to school.

I was interested, therefore, in some comments made by girls who had been lured into enrolling in the special classes even though initially they resisted the idea.

1 They told me about the Teen Mother Program. I didn't really want to go there, but I said, "Well, what's the harm in checking it out?" So I went and checked it, and I found that I *liked* it there. So—believe it or not—a year later I graduated! I had earned all my credits at the Teen Mother Program, and I knew everything there was to know about childbirth—I learned it from them—and all about birth control, all about taking care of a baby.

2 Well, see—when I first found out I was pregnant, I didn't want to go to school. Then my cousin was attending this special

class, and she told me how it was and stuff—all the things they teach you, and you could make things for the baby. And that made me *want* to go to school. So I went there, and did pretty good there. Better than what I did at any of the other schools.

Since almost all the girls I talked with had attended one of the special classes during pregnancy, it seemed important to find out what effect these programs had had upon them. They often started talking about the classes before I had even mentioned them, and their remarks focused on four principal topics: the close association among class members, the curriculum, the teachers, and their own accomplishments.

Many remarked about the common bond that enabled girls who might otherwise never have become acquainted to form a close, supportive fellowship at a time of mutual need, and to participate willingly in classroom activities.

1 I met a lot of people that were in the same condition, which I think helped a *lot.* I know it did. Because I didn't feel like I was the only one. I knew other people in the same circumstances, and I felt better. I didn't feel so alone.

2 That place is the best school that I have ever seen in my life. To be a girl like I was—pregnant and nowhere to turn—I really didn't know I had a place to turn. And I went there, and I was so scared because I didn't know anybody, and even then, seeing another young teen-ager pregnant, I thought, "Oh, look at her! Isn't it a shame—all these young girls?" And then I thought, "Look at me. I'm here. I'm here, too."

The curriculum provided instruction designed to prepare the girls for childbirth, and information about infant care, child development, and family planning, along with the usual academic classes.

1 Everything I wanted to know about babies, about going to the hospital, about pregnancy—I learned there.

2 We had sex education, she explained all that. She had a whole bunch of books we could look at and find out about it. She'd

just sit down and talk to us. She said, "Whatever you want to know, just ask me, and I'll help you."

But it was the teachers that the girls talked about most. At times when they felt rejected by parents or boy friends, or when they were depressed or confused, it was these teachers they turned to. This was expressed so well by Jenifer, who had gone through an especially lonely, difficult time during pregnancy.

I think that the only thing that was a bright point, was the class. Because I knew if I had a fight with Howie, or what have you, I could always come to my teacher and cry at her about it.

If I'd had to go to a regular school, I don't think I would have made it, because there were times when the baby would be up all night, or something would have happened where I wouldn't have gotten an assignment done, and a regular teacher would have just said, "Well, you put yourself in that predicament—now you'll just have to live with it." Whereas my teacher was able to understand. She didn't let us get away with murder, but she was able to let us kind of go at a pace that was comfortable for us. I don't think I would have graduated without her.

Any attempt to measure the effectiveness of a particular teacher requires an assessment of the quantity and quality of learning achieved by the students. Many of the girls had had both attendance problems and learning problems in their traditional schools, yet some expressed the pride they felt in their accomplishments in the special classes, and in so doing drew some comparisons between different methods of teaching.

I never learned so much in my life—I'll put it that way. The teacher was the greatest teacher I ever had. She would help you.

See, a lot of teachers—I mean, they don't really take the time to sit down and help you. They don't take the time to have, like, special things to discuss and talk about. They give you outlines, tell you to go home and do this, and do this. They don't really ... I'm sure they would if you asked them—but who's going to ask them?

Without motivation on the part of the student to learn, however, even the best teaching can be ineffective. Lucia's comments are interesting because they trace her lagging progress from irresponsibility to self motivation.

Well, to tell you the truth, I think if I hadn't got pregnant, I probably would have never finished school. Because I was really terrible in school. I used to always get in trouble and not go, and they kicked me out two or three times. I was just really terrible. But then, when I transferred to the special class, they helped you more, you know, it was just easier to do, and I went there for the whole last year. And I feel if I hadn't gone over there I would never have graduated.

Why do you think you were goofing off so much in high school?

Oh, I don't know, I just didn't like school. It was a hassle, it was hard for me. I wasn't that good in it. It was easier just to stay home, not get out of bed, or to run off with my friends and go to a party, or—you know—anything just to get out of school. It was just a hassle.

Didn't your mother want you to go to school?

Definitely!

Was this something that you fought about a lot?

Sometimes ... well, at first we did. Then it just got to the point where she wasn't going to say anything about it.

You're the youngest in the family. Did she sort of give up on you?

Yeah, you could say that.

What did you think you could do with your life? What were your plans?

I didn't have any. There was nothing.

When I first started going to the special class, I started messing off, and I wasn't even going. So it was the same old thing all over again—just not even going, not getting out of bed.

Then the teacher talked to my mom, and she told my mom that if I didn't start going and everything, I wasn't going to get my credits, I wasn't—you know— going to graduate. My mom just talked to me, and I told her, "Yeah, yeah! Okay, okay! I'll go, I'll go!"—you know.

And I started going, you know, once or twice . . . and then I just made up my mind, decided I was going to go because I wanted to graduate—because nobody thought I could do it. I didn't think I could do it, and then I did it—I graduated! I started going regularly, I got all my work caught up. Like second semester, I had finished all my work for the whole semester in one month. Nobody could believe it. I was doing fantastic!

For girls who did not complete requirements for graduation while attending the special class, the time inevitably came when they had to go back to regular high school. Some made the transfer successfully, some chose to go to adult school instead, and others, like Charmaine, returned to high school but soon dropped out. She found she had outgrown her former girl friends, who "wanted to be out in the street waving at guys," and she said her teachers "wouldn't spend time" with her. Of her experience in the special class she remarked, "I wished that I could go to that class without having to be pregnant."

Those that persevered to the finish, and received their high school diplomas at commencement exercises, expressed pride in their accomplishment. And they remembered the circumstances very well.

I graduated! I was still pregnant—I was two weeks overdue when I graduated—and I went down the ramp and the whole bit. I couldn't believe it!

At the time of the interviews, 52 of the 126 girls had already completed high school, and 44 more showed firm intentions of doing so. The others—30 in number—had either dropped out, or seemed unmotivated to complete the requirements.

Some of those who had dropped out spoke of their plans to complete high school, and maybe even go on to college. But they kept talking about how hard it was to do this, now that they had a child. I asked Dolly, for instance, who was in the tenth grade, whether she was attending school regularly, and her reply was, "Yes, when the baby's not sick. But she's been sick the last month and a half."

Lack of adequate child care was their hardest problem. While some girls were able to take advantage of a child care center provided by local schools, colleges, or churches, many others had to depend on their families for help. And sometimes a family's patience wore thin.

I don't go no more. I went all this year, except I stopped about four months ago. I was supposed to graduate this year. See, my mom was complaining about baby sitting and this and that, so I just stopped.

I always said through the whole thing, I said I wasn't going to quit, but then I ended up quitting anyways. Now I have to wait until the baby gets older to go to college, probably won't even be able to carry out a career—now. I think it would be too hard.

On the other hand, as time went by, some girls who had dropped out of high school and had some job experience began to take a fresh look at education. Regina was twenty-one when I saw her, a widow with a four-year-old child. She had been employed in a hospital as a housekeeper, and had liked the job and the people she worked with. But all of a sudden—she even remembered the day!—she made the big decision to go back to school and earn a diploma.

One Saturday I just told myself, "I'm not going to go back there to make any more beds or clean up any more." I said to myself, "I'm going to go to school, I'm going to get up there. I'm by myself now, I'm going to have to do the best I can for me and my boy." So that's what I'm doing—I'm doing it right now.

People say you don't need a high school diploma, you know. I've run across people saying, "You don't need it, they never ask you for a diploma." But now, it seems to me you can't get a good job without a good education—a good job, you know, with money—and I'm talking about—not a little, you know, not the minimum wages. I want a *lot* of money—who doesn't? But that's why I'm going to school now—so I can better myself. And make a lot of money!

CHAPTER TWELVE

Attitudes toward the Church

Since the church has a centuries-old tradition of "ministering" to those who turn to it for help, it seemed appropriate to find out from the girls who were interviewed whether the church had been helpful to them. There was no intent to explore their religious beliefs or inquire into their church preferences, but rather to find out if they had turned to the church—*any* church—as a potential source of help during a difficult period in their lives, or whether the church—*any* church—during that same period had reached out to them.

It should be remembered that during the early period of pregnancy the girls were faced by the necessity of reaching certain decisions that would affect the rest of their lives. Then, after their children were born, they had to come to grips with more decisions, none of them easy. Some girls had been rebuffed by parents or boy friends, and were feeling more and more lonely. As they watched some old dreams fade, they had to begin to reshape their lives, and take a long, long look into the future.

Many of the girls brought up the subject of the church on their own initiative. If they did not, discussion was invited by a simple question, "Is the church important to you?"

Responses varied widely, as might be expected. A few were brief and expressed negative feelings, such as, "We're not religious at all," which effectively closed off further discussion of the subject. But most girls wanted to talk about experiences they had had, and they expressed their views about the church quite freely, and often went on to discuss their own religious beliefs.

Each story in this chapter describes a particular situation: how a certain girl, when she was experiencing serious problems, felt about a certain church, its priest or pastor, or its members. She may well have been feeling hurt and angry when she walked through the church door—the anger stemming from the desertion of her boy friend, perhaps, or the rejection of her parents. She may have brought with her a heavy sense of frustration and anguish over what seemed to her a twist of fate—"Why did this happen to *me?*"

The significant point is that many of the girls did turn to the church when their spirits were low. Did they find comfort and help? Did they feel welcome? When they needed someone to talk to, was anybody there? Did they seek the blessing of the church for their marriage, or the baptism of their children? While discussing topics of this nature, some of the girls talked about their own personal religious beliefs and doubts, their hopes and disappointments, and their search for the kind of church they wanted.

The ties to church were very strong in Charlotte's case. When she turned to it for spiritual comfort, she found it, and she felt the church members provided welcome support.

> My mother brought us up in the church. When I was pregnant, I had a lot of confusions, and I was constantly upset with my boy friend. Everything he did or said upset me real bad, and I just couldn't deal with it. I would just cry and cry and cry. Then I started going to church, and I would just pray for the Lord to help me, and I overcame those things and they just don't bother me any more.
>
> Everybody there was real good. They offered to help with everything.
>
> I don't know what some churches could do, but I know our church—if there is a problem, they'll sit down and talk to you. If it's a real big problem, they'll offer to help you out with that—you know, financially. Or if it's just counseling—someone you need to talk to, and work it out with—they'll sit and talk to you. Our church really helps. I don't know too much about other churches ... but our church helps.

Harriet also had a good, warm feeling about her church. When she was going through a particularly difficult time in her life, she felt shored up by people who had known her since she was a little girl.

I was raised in church. The people at church—the minister, you know, and everybody—really helped me a lot. They were behind me, and if I was down I could talk to one of them, you know. It really, really helped. I mean, a lot of times I didn't even have to seek help out. I didn't have to ... they just—they knew, you know. Because, like I said, I'm going to the same church that I've been going to since I was about five, and they know me, you know. If I'm down, they can tell just by talking to me on the phone. And they were really good to me, they were really a big help when I needed them.

But some of the girls said they felt a little less than welcome at church. It is possible, of course, that the criticism they felt was more imaginary than real. The important thing is that they *felt* they were being scrutinized, and it bothered them.

I go to church ... well, the church is kind of far, it's on the other side of the tracks ... so I go whenever I can get up early enough to go, or when there is nothing to do ... But when I do go—I don't know—I feel kind of like—people stare at you. *Why do you feel that they stare at you?*
Because first of all, I don't have a ring, I'm not married yet. I look so young to have a baby, you know. I take her with me. I'm not ashamed, I could care less what people think, because me myself ... I always thought, you know ... people talk, it's going to hit them back, someone in their family is going to have the same problem, you know, they ain't got nothing more to say ... Like my aunt—she was always telling my mom, "Your daughter is disgusting!"—yet her daughter got pregnant when she was twelve years old. You see? It always hits someone back, you know, when they start saying stuff like that ... So, it doesn't bother me. I just go, you know, and sit there. My little girl, she acts real good in church, and then when we come out, we just take the bus home.

Gretchen talked about the church of her childhood with a certain nostalgia that may have been associated in her mind with a simpler, happier, less complex time in her life. But when she drew a comparison between that church and other churches she had attended, she put her finger on the factor that made the biggest difference to her.

When I was in Missouri, I was going to church and I was in a church group and everything. I enjoyed it a lot. But when I came out here I tried to ... I went back to church for a while, but it just wasn't the same thing.

I was in a small town there, 250 people, and everyone was close, and when I came out here, it was kind of impersonal ... I just couldn't get back into it. Well, they're friendly and everything at the churches here, but back there they made you feel more comfortable, you know.

When Wilma was asked, "Is the church important to you?" she replied with feeling, "Yes, I *love* church! It's just something in me. I like to go to church." She described her devotion to the church in Arkansas, and the church she attended after she came to California. Then her mood changed, and she revealed the hurt she felt, but couldn't express, except in angry criticism of the church.

In Arkansas I was just going to church every Sunday, every Sunday. They have church like all day Sunday. I'd be right there. I used to read the Bible, I used to stay with it. Then, when I moved out here, my first year that I was out here, I was really into church, too.

I don't even go to that church any more. I look around, I just go from different churches to different churches.
What are you looking for in a church?
Okay now ... I was going to this church ... if you walk in there, they look you up and down ... "What is she doing here?" ... and stuff like that. And that ain't the way to be going to church—somebody look you up and down—you be going there to serve the Lord and not them. And they act like you're coming there to serve *them*. I don't like that. I think they just should ... it's a shame how most churches is now ... I wouldn't be going to serve them no way—I don't care how

they look at me—I be going just to listen to the service and stuff like that ... because I don't really care about what other peoples think.

Do you want your little girl to go to church?

Yes, I would like her to. Because I miss going to church and singing in the choirs and everything.

Several girls described how they felt accepted and welcome in certain church groups that go by the general name, "Christians." Rena said that she and her boy friend "go to church about three times a week," though neither one had ever had much previous church experience.

We're both Christians now. And it's pretty important to us.

It was about five months ago. Casey hurt himself, and he couldn't work. Since he couldn't work, we couldn't pay the rent. So we called the Hotline. We told them we didn't have any place to live and we didn't have any money. So we stayed with these people, and they were Christians. They never forced anything on us—like the meetings they'd go to—but they'd talk about it once in a while. He was never mean to her or anything. They never argued—I'm sure they had their little disagreements—but they never argued, and they told us to save all our money and get our own place. They wouldn't let us buy food or pay them for staying there.

Only a few girls referred to counseling services provided by the church. During the early period of pregnancy, when they were consumed by doubts and fears, they were far more likely to unburden themselves to their friends than to parents, pastor, or priest. To be sure, two or three girls described family conferences involving pastors, at which plans for early marriage were discussed; but these events could be considered "counseling" sessions only in a limited sense, for the pastor was simply endorsing a decision that had already been reached, and facilitating action on it.

Although it was very difficult for most girls to initiate any discussion of their pregnancy with an adult, that does not necessarily mean they would have resisted all attempts by sensitive counselors to reach out to them with an offer of help. Rosemary expressed her feelings in this regard.

> I was raised a Catholic. I was baptized, confirmed, got my first holy communion, went to parochial school—everything.
>
> And my mother went to her friend who is a priest, who was a very good friend of hers, and she was all upset. And he said, "Well, you just have to thank God that she didn't abort the baby."
>
> But he never tried to get a hold of me to talk to me about it—nothing.
>
> So I haven't gone to church since then. I figure, you know, they're supposed to be the people who are there for you when you need them, and when I needed them the most, I didn't feel that I could go to them. And seeing that the one priest was such a good friend of the family, I figured he would come to me, and he never did.
>
> I had my children both baptized Catholics, but I won't force them to go, because of my feelings. I just can't go.

Ellen never forgot the experience she had had when she was fourteen and pregnant. Unlike Rosemary, she decided to *ask* for help. The church had been an important part of her life, and she had gone to a particular church for eight years. "I was really into church," she said. "I mean, it was Sunday nights, Sunday mornings, Wednesday nights—I mean, every church day, I was the Good Book all over again." When she realized she was pregnant, it seemed natural to her to consult her minister. Her mother agreed this was a good plan, and drove her to the church.

> Now you have to understand that I was very scared. I went to him asking him for help. He was the one I felt closest to. I stated that I was pregnant, I didn't know what to do, I didn't know where to turn. I was in there for two hours, and I told him the whole story about my boyfriend and myself. And he says, "Well, come back and see me tomorrow." And when I came back—I had not talked to him about anything else except

that I was pregnant—he stated, "Come back when you don't have your problem any more."

I had felt he was sympathetic—the way he looked. But then when he gave me his answer, I figured that he didn't even think about it, that he just thought, "Well, she played around, that's against the Lord," you know, "she's a sinner. I don't want her in my church." The way he looked at me—like I wasn't, I just wasn't the right "church material."

It shattered everything I thought about the church.

There were other times in their lives besides the period of pregnancy when the girls felt a need for special help with a problem. Jane, for example, went through a very bad time after the birth of her child. She was searching for an "answer," and she turned to the church.

I went to a counselor at our church who helped me get over a lot of things that I couldn't get over myself. This was about a year ago, to be exact. Because I could not handle it ... Sure, I have desires—like now, I have desires—but it doesn't go to the point where I go and do it. That's not my idea. I thought I could get love just by going to bed.

I could talk to this counselor about anything. She is available at all times. She comes over here, or I go to the church. She just says, "Well, meet me at the church, or I'll come over there." And I say, "Okay—fine."

My mom ... she was going to leave my dad so many times when he was drinking ... because he'd come home drunk ... And my mom just stuck with it and prayed, and stuck with it ... and she got her answer. Now I want mine.

Many of the girls—including some who had had no church connection previously—wanted very much to be married in a church. This usually necessitated the fulfillment of certain requirements—premarital counseling by a clergyman, or attendance at a series of marriage preparation classes, or both. The personality of the minister or priest often seemed as important to the young people as his counsel.

We always go to church—even before we were married, we'd go every Sunday. And when we found out I was pregnant, we went and talked to the pastor, and he was just so nice. He asked us, "Is there any reason ... ?" We had planned not to tell him that I was pregnant. And he asked us if there was any other reason why we wanted to get married—and you can't sit there and lie in front of the minister. I just looked at Craig and kind of giggled, and we told him. He was really nice.

He told us, "Any time you guys get into a big hairy fight, just give me a call on the phone." But he did tell us, "Take a walk together each night, even if it's just across the street to Betsy Ross, or around the block, by yourselves. Get the next-door neighbor to come watch the baby for fifteen minutes. Because that's really good—it gives you a chance to talk."
That sounds like good advice.

It is. We never do it, but it's good advice.

In Juanita's story, feelings of disappointment and rejection, when original marriage plans could not be carried out, led her and her young husband to explore other possibilities, and eventually to start a new church life in a completely different setting.

At the time I was Catholic, and Victor wasn't baptized into anything, so to get married through the Catholic church you have to go through classes in a six-week period, and I thought, "Gee! That's too long to wait!" Then, when they found out I was pregnant, they said, "No, you can't get married here."
Was this the priest in your own parish who said this?

Yeah. We went to talk to him, and my mom did, too, and he said, "No," because it's against the Catholic standards or something, and that you have to be holy and pure, you know, when you get married. So—I really felt bad, you know—that made me feel worse, and my mom said we could get married at City Hall. I guess when you're younger you think you have to get married in this big old wedding, and not through City Hall.

So then my husband's best friend said, "You know, we got

married through this minister. Why don't you try him?" So we called him, and he was really nice and understanding, and he said, "Yes," we could rent out the church and it would only be twenty dollars. And he said, "Just tell me the day, and we'll set it all up," and he was really nice. From time to time he'll talk to us, you know. He knows we have two kids now.

What kind of church do you go to now?

We go to a Pentecostal church. It's nearby, and it's very helpful to us. They have a nursery school for our little boy and he goes there, and he really likes it. Victor has a men's group, and every Saturday they have like a fellowship breakfast, and it's free and all the men go. And then I'm in the Women's Club, and we fix lunches, and we raise money. We do different crafts, and we help out, you know—we make baskets for Easter. It's really nice! I like it, and all the people are so nice, and they help you out—anything you need, I mean, they're right there.

Do you feel as though people care about you?

Yeah. Because, when I got pregnant, I thought, "Oh man! I'm really going to go to Hell now, because I did this!" But these people give you the satisfaction—like, not everybody's perfect. Everybody has that little black dot in their heart, everybody has something in their soul, I guess, that they're not proud of, and—like now, I'm not ashamed that I got pregnant. I really am not.

From several accounts, it appeared that when girls were denied the privilege of being married in a particular church, they simply turned to another church, or were married in a civil ceremony.

When they wanted to have their babies baptized, however, there was only one place to go. They had to obtain the blessing of the church.

Those who were unmarried when they approached the church regarding baptism for their child met with varying reactions. When I asked one of the girls whether the fact that they were not married had posed any problem when she and the baby's father asked to have their child baptized, she made this reply.

> They, like ... well, kind of. They kind of like said that they don't like to do it with people that aren't married. And he goes, that he hopes that we get married, you know. He talked with us for a while, and ... but they still did it.

Another unmarried girl had found it very easy to talk with the priests about her child's baptism, even though she had to take care of this alone.

> Yeah, they were real nice. They knew I wasn't married and everything, but they had nothing against it. It was one more person to worship God, so you know, they're happy about it. I plan to convert Tim one of these days. Hopefully.

Married girls indicated they felt the baptizing of a child was a matter for both parents to think about and to decide upon jointly. For some it was important to have the child baptized at a very early age. Others were less sure what they wanted to do, and decided to postpone it.

> My husband wants him to have his freedom in religion—to be able to choose. He doesn't want him baptized until he knows what he wants to be, because he might want to be something entirely different.

And in the following instance, the girl went along with her husband's wishes, but said she would have preferred to delay this decision.

> We did have him baptized. I really didn't want to, you know. My husband wanted him to, and everybody else, so I said, "All right." I myself think it is his choice to make. I would have rather waited until he was seven or eight, and let him decide what church *he* wanted to go to, *whether* he wanted to go, and if he wanted to be baptized in a certain denomination or whatever.

Although some girls who had been brought up in the church

continued the habits of their childhood and attended church regularly, others said they had stopped going. Maria was one of those who had dropped out, and as she talked, a wistful quality could be detected in some of her remarks.

Oh, when I was young, yeah, I always used to go to church. *All* the time we used to go to church ... And then, right after I was pregnant I was going, really going to church, and praying.

I think it's nice. If you're in the mood to go to church ... waking up, being dressed all nice, taking a shower, dressing up your baby, and going to church ...

Sometimes they talk interesting. I remember they used to talk about what's going on in the world right now, about husbands, wives, mothers, sins, all this ... Sometimes they really talk interesting, you know, when they talk about God, how it was ... and just things like that. Sometimes they would talk interesting, and sometimes they wouldn't.

But—it's a hassle, walking down the street when it's hot and stuff. It's better when you have a car and you go—like it's hard for me, you know. I don't go to church any more at all.

Rita, on the other hand, had had no church upbringing, and felt she had missed something. Now seventeen, with a two-year-old child, she was trying to keep house for her father and the younger children since the death of her mother.

Church? I don't really go to church. I probably would go if I didn't have so many problems. I feel like I need a lot of help right now, and I don't have time to go to church. I don't know. I don't really think that it helps me, because I haven't went. I've never tried it, but I don't know if it would help.

My family believe in God and all this, but they don't never attend church. My mom was one of these types—pray, pray, praying—all the time. My dad isn't, but my mom was.
Did your family have you go to classes in the church?

Yes, when we were young—but even those classes I ditched. So I never finished ... See, that's why my older sister lived a whole different life, because she had to go to classes, she made her first holy communion, she made her confirmation. She had to do everything, because my mom sent her to church, she had to go to those classes. With us, she started like letting go of us. My sister's doing real good, and I wish—I think sometimes I wish she would have took care of me that way. I wish she would have held me back that way.

Are you saying the church has helped your sister?

Yeah. I think it has, because she was more of a real—I think—more decent girl. Even now, she still goes to church. She sends her little girl to church, and her little girl already made her first holy communion. Her little girl's seven ... My sister's a whole different person, you know.

A few girls spoke of having feelings of guilt because they had had a child out of wedlock. One of them was Hilda, who had been reared in the Catholic church and felt strong ties to it. Though she was bothered at times by some nagging worries and unanswered questions, she remained faithful to her church and derived strength from her own personal beliefs.

I need to brush up on my religion really bad. There's a lot of things I don't understand. We go to church every Sunday—I've always gone to church every Sunday—and I take the baby with me. But it's just that there's a lot of things that I don't understand ...

Like, they said I should have gone to confession and confessed. I still haven't done that, because I think when you confess it, you're saying, like, you're sorry. And I didn't think it was a sin—so I haven't confessed it. My mother told me, she said, "Oh, you haven't even gone to confession and told the priest anything about it?" And I said, "No, I haven't."

Then, too, I don't know, I guess I need to learn more about my religion. Because maybe it *is* wrong that me and my boyfriend live together, and I have her ... and then we get up on Sunday morning and go to church. He enjoys going, because it's something we can do together. We just get up now on Sundays and go.

I just ... I say my prayers. I believe in God, you know. So I always say my prayers to keep the baby healthy and whatever. And I feel like I really depend on Him to protect me. I really depend on God a lot. You know, like when I leave the baby with the baby sitter, I worry so much, and I just pray that she's okay, pray that I make it home to pick her up.

Several girls, on the other hand, had rejected altogether any connection with an established church. They took pains, however, to make a clear distinction between their feelings about the church, and their feelings about God. As one girl put it: "Church in general, no. God and the Bible, yes."

This predilection for personalized religious beliefs was illustrated time and time again through comments the girls volunteered when talking about the church. For example, Sabrina, who had been reared in a fundamentalist church by a church-going family, blamed "the people at churches" for making her avoid them altogether. She launched a bitter attack on church members—and then expounded on her own unconventional concept of God.

> They're nothing but a bunch of hypocrites. They claim not to do this, and not to do that, and tell me that I'm sinful, "You'll die and go to Hell!"—and they turn right around and do it theirself.
>
> I have my own belief, and my own feelings, and I feel God's very liberated—I really do—and that, you know, He don't *expect* us to live like they did back in Adam and Eve. He just don't *expect* that of us, and I just feel that He's really liberated and understands the way things are today. That's why I don't talk about religion! I just know that God's there. I talk to Him all the time.

And Jeannette reserved the right to question the stand her church had taken in a matter that concerned her own values.

Before we got married we discussed birth control, and my husband was all for no birth control, because we're Christians, and we believe more or less that if God blesses us to be able to afford children, then we will have children. But I was kind of shaky on it, and I said—well, I didn't want to say that maybe God would make a mistake—but I didn't want to take any chances either. I wanted some method of birth control.

In spite of doubts and anxieties about the role of the church in their lives, there were some girls who really wanted to find a church where they could feel at home, where there was someone they could turn to for help, and people that made them feel wanted. And some were actively seeking such a church. No one more than Jodie.

I'd like to find a nice church that has a sermon and everything, but I'd like it to be where you could *talk* to the priest. Because all the ones I've been to, they don't really talk to you—they shake your hand at the door, and that's it. And I'd want a place where you could go up and you could say, "Hey, I've got a problem. Can I talk to you now?" And have the person listen and help you out.

And even if they just had group sessions, like some churches do—and you could just talk to other people about your kids and things. Because when you go to church you don't get time to meet anybody. You just go in and sit down and listen. It's *hard* —because you've got some things you need help with.

But I can't find no good church to go to, though. I'm going to try a Lutheran next week. It might be nice. I'm not sure.

CHAPTER THIRTEEN

Advice to Others

The wide range of topics discussed during each interview, and the intensity of feeling which certain subjects evoked, had allowed little opportunity for the girls to take a long look at what had happened in their lives and see it with any degree of perspective. It seemed important to provide such an opportunity, for they had all been through an experience which had completely reshaped their lives. A short time earlier they had been children, and now they were all parents. Whereas most people take time for the orderly progression from childhood to adolescence, and from adolescence to maturity, these young mothers had had to take the giant step from childhood to maturity without the cushion, the comfort, the luxury of adolescence.

Accordingly, each girl was asked to think back over what had happened during the past several years, or months, and to consider what effect these events had had upon her as a person. How did she feel about having had a child so early in life? What, if anything, would she do differently if she had it to do over again? What advice would she give someone else?

When asked how they felt about becoming mothers at such an early age, many girls revealed a great deal of ambivalence. On the one hand, they loved their children very much; on the other hand, they had never worked so hard in their lives.

> Oh, I've really enjoyed it. It's really neat! It's hard, I wish I would have waited, but I'm happy that I have her, you know ... there would be nothing that I would ... I would never give her up, you know.
>
> Once in a long while I feel ... oh, why did I get pregnant? I'm still young, you know! But I'm really happy with her ... it's hard, it really is hard—especially when you're young—it's hard.

On two points there was virtually unanimous agreement: having a child had *made* them grow up; and, it had been *hard*. The girl who had her first child when she was only twelve made this comment.

> There were so many times that I was ready just to give up. At twelve years old you're just a kid yourself. They said, "A kid raising a kid." They still tell me that now, but they don't think of me as a kid any more.
> *You've done a lot of growing up in a short time, haven't you?*
> The hard way!

It had been hard for a number of reasons. For instance, it was a shock to discover that the daily routine of a mother is rather limited. As one girl remarked, "It all seems so rosy when you're looking at it, you know—from the other side." An eighteen-year-old girl frankly admitted she was tired taking care of her child, who was at the time of the interview not quite six months old.

> After I had the baby I started getting tired of taking care of him. Now that I'm living at Kurt's house, there's a lot of people, and all day long they take care of him, and once in a while I'll take care of him. But I think if I lived in an apartment and Kurt was at work, and it was just me and the baby, that I'd probably be a nervous wreck, because I really don't like responsibility.
> When I had to take care of the baby for six weeks by myself, there were a lot of times I was going crazy. I was getting tired of taking care of him, and I wanted to go out to parties and stuff. I didn't like the responsibility. I just wanted to go out when I wanted, and I couldn't, because I had the baby.

They also stressed the fact that they had missed out on so many good times, and so many experiences that most teen-agers enjoy.

> I missed out on quite a bit. I never went to a prom, and oh, when I see the girls getting ready to go to the proms now I think, "Gee! I wish this hadn't happened!" ... I'm glad it happened, but I look back and I see everything that I missed.

Sixteen years old, and you've got your whole life ahead of you! You know—you miss out on the parties, the proms, the football games—you just miss out on a lot. I didn't realize just how much I would be missing out on, till I missed it all.

It had been difficult, too, for a girl to have to concentrate on the needs of a child before she had had time to decide what she wanted out of life for herself.

I really didn't know where I was at, at that time. I hadn't gotten myself sorted out, I hadn't decided where my life was heading, or what my thoughts were. I was very confused. Then all of a sudden—here, before I had myself figured out, I've got a kid to figure out! And before I could really be responsible for myself, I'm responsible for somebody else. And it's really a hard thing.

Severe limitations on personal freedom, lost opportunities for fun and good times with their friends, and the burden of responsibility for another person at a time when their own identity had not yet been established—those were some of the costs of growing up by the method they had chosen: having a child.

Some of those who had been especially rebellious, experimenting with one thrill after another, actually credited their early motherhood with rescuing them from a destructive way of life. They were convinced that pregnancy had "put the brakes on them" when all else had failed. Jamie spoke for these girls when she made the following remarks.

If I would have went the same route I was going, and I wouldn't have gotten pregnant, I would have turned out bad. I'd probably be over in Las Vegas making money the wrong way—this is how I was. Because I was rebelling. I was getting love the wrong way—at least I thought it was love. I know myself I would have turned out bad, because I wouldn't have cared. I was getting to the point that I didn't care.

It made me mature *fast*. It cut off a lot, but at the same time it did quite a lot for me, because my son made me realize that— "Hey! It's time to grow up!" you know. "If you keep playing around ... you're going into a woman now, you've got to change!" Otherwise, I'd probably be playing fifteen-year-old games yet, you know, and with him I *have* to grow up.

The sobering effect which having a child had had upon these young mothers was evident. Most were quick to assert that they had grown up, though when I asked Jamie if she felt the price had been rather high, she responded, "Yes! *Very high!*"

A few of the girls freely admitted that the process of growing up was far from complete. A girl of nineteen, with a two-year-old child, made this cautious assessment when she was asked if it had been a good experience or not for her to have a child so early in life.

I feel like it was half good and half bad. It's made me grow up a lot—a lot, you know; but then, it was bad, because in a lot of ways I haven't—still haven't grown up, you know. I can't really explain it.

Of course, just how competent and grown up they really felt no doubt varied from day to day or, as in Gail's case, from crisis to crisis. She had been working very hard to help her husband combat alcoholism, and so, when considered in that context, it was not a simple matter to say whether having a child to care for had been a good experience or not.

Now, since everything's happened ... *now* I can say, "I think it's good." But if you would have asked me this a couple of months ago, I would have said, "It's rotten!" But I think it's good ... it's hard—it's harder than I ever imagined—but it's good.

As they grew accustomed to their new feelings of maturity and responsibility, they discovered that their ability to form good judgments had improved remarkably—especially regarding men. This inevitably caused some of the unmarried girls to examine their relationships with the boys who were the fathers of their children, and to decide whether or not to continue these relationships. Andrea, for example, whose child was then a year old, felt the time had come for a firm understanding with her boy friend.

I told him that we're going to get things straightened out soon, because I'm not going to be waiting around. I have to get *going,* you know! I can't stay here with my sister all the time—there's things I have to do, and it would be harder for me if he's just playing a game with me, saying that we're going to go back and me keeping my hopes up, and we're not. I told him that either he's serious about it, or why not let me know now, because there's things I have to plan. And if we don't work out, I want to move away from here so I can forget him—because it's going to be hard.

With increased self confidence had come increased self respect. This was an important factor with many of the single girls in their relationships with men on a dating basis.

I've been out with a couple of guys that, since I've had a man, have tried everything in the book—being nice, or going ahead and attacking you, or whatever. And I say, "Look! If that's the way you want it, just take me home." And a couple just haven't even talked to me any more.

You can't do something like that—you hold no respect for yourself—that's the way I feel. And just because I had a kid doesn't mean that I don't have any respect.

It was one thing to have grown up, and to feel as if they had some control over their lives, and were better able to make choices than they had been before they had a child. But if they could somehow turn back the clock to the time before they became pregnant, would they do anything differently?

A few—very, very few—said they would not. One of the older girls, who had been married at seventeen and felt happy and contented with her husband and three children, expressed the feelings of this small minority when she said, "No, no. I wouldn't. I wouldn't do it any different."

A few others, also married, rationalized that having children so early in life might actually have some advantages, allowing them to look forward to carefree days to come—compensation, perhaps, for that desirable adolescence they had missed?

> Having our children so young and being happy with our life the way it is, we'll still be young when they go out on their own, and then we can do the things that we really want to do—travel, and so forth—and really enjoy ourselves.

Most of the girls, however, said they would act quite differently in certain respects if they could live part of their lives over again. In the first place, they would get to know a boy friend very, very well before they risked having a child by him. In a great many cases the girls no longer cared for the father of the child, and in certain instances felt extremely bitter toward him. There had been violent incidents, even among those who had married the father, and some marriages had already ended in separation or divorce.

One of the youngest girls, who was only fourteen when she had her baby, made it very clear that she regretted ever having become involved with the father of her child.

> Well, one thing I wish I would have done is get to know him better. And I don't mean, you know, know him for three months, or know him for three years—I mean get to know him inside and outside, and know what he thinks and how he feels. And then—birth control!

Another conclusion many girls had reached was that it had been a serious mistake not to get to know a number of boys before they settled on one particular boy exclusively. One of the married girls admitted, "Sometimes I get the itches to go out and just meet other guys, which is hurting our marriage," and another made the following comment.

> I wouldn't get tied down with one boy and not go out with anyone else. 'Cause that's what happened to me. I just liked Bert, and I just wanted to be with him. But if I could do it over again, I think I would date a *lot* of boys—as many boys as I could—and different kinds of boys. You know—boys from

different ways. And finish school. And then maybe think about getting married — *then*.

In addition, there were the poignant comments of girls who had finally found a man they really loved, and wished they had waited for him.

I wish now that I could give this person, who is so special to me, who means so much more to me than anybody else ever has ... I wish I could give him all the things I gave to Alan before I ended up with a baby. There are so many things that I would love for him to have, that I would love to be able to give him ... just picking up somewhere and taking off, or going out just whenever I feel like it, and not have to worry about coming home too late to put the baby in bed, and have somebody to take care of him, you know ... all those things. I don't feel cheated, but I feel like I am cheating him ... Oh, I can't believe it! Like I said, I can't believe I ever settled for anything less than this.

Of special interest also were some thoughtful comments made by girls who had come to realize they were not at all ready to have a child when they did, and wished they had waited much longer. Cory, for instance, had just been saying how important she thought it was for girls to know about birth control, and how she intended to inform her own daughter and also tell her all about what she had gone through. Since she had spoken with real feeling, I asked her to be more explicit.

Well, I wasn't ready for a child. I had no idea what a responsibility it was going to be — especially having a sick child. I wasn't emotionally ready for it, and I'm still not. It's been almost five years since I had her, and if I would have known then what I know now, I don't think I would have even wanted to start a family yet.

I had had a lot of trouble at home, and I think I was running away from my parents when I met my husband. And actually I ran away from a situation *into* a situation. It was hard on both of us, me and my husband, raising a child. He had had his freedom before, and I don't think he was ready to settle down ... And there's so many things you have to go through day by day. You have to spend your time together, and spend your time with your child, and it's just ... I had no time for *anything* else. It caused a lot of problems between us.

There were times when I just felt like I couldn't take it any more, and I had to yell and scream at somebody. Luckily, Bruce is the type, that I could yell and scream at him, and he'd just take it in his stride and tell me, "Now calm down!" and he'd take the baby and take over ... So I just wasn't ready ... at that time.

If I could have the same child that I do now, I would have waited quite a bit longer to have one.

A great many girls would have agreed with Cory's sentiments. If they had it to do over again—they would have *waited*. And thinking back over the events of the past few years, they were able to identify the principal reasons why they had *not* waited, but instead had allowed themselves to be propelled into a responsibility for which they had no preparation, and in some cases, no desire.

Their biggest problem had been lack of information. "If I had only known!" was a phrase I was to hear time and time again. Some girls had had virtually no information about sex—they did not, for example, comprehend the nature of sexual intercourse. A great many had critical gaps in their knowledge, as evidenced by the girl who said, "I didn't know that you could get pregnant so *fast.*"

Had their parents talked with them about sex, and answered whatever questions they had? Only a few said they had. Far more said that sex was never discussed in their homes because parents would not allow it. Some who thought their parents might have been willing to talk with them under better circumstances, were feeling so alienated from their parents at that particular time that they simply could not approach them on such a sensitive matter as sex. In other situations, parents were just too busy to spend time with their children, and so the children felt they had to find things out for themselves.

> My mom and dad were always just too busy for me. They never took time to teach me what sex was. All us girls had to learn it ... Thank God we're all right now, because there was a time when all of us were rotten. You wouldn't even *want* to be our mother! ... And my mom and dad were just too busy for us. We had to learn everything ourselves. Everything.

Some parents had tried to give their daughters basic information about sex and reproduction, but had either left out important elements, or had failed to use language the girls could understand. One of them said she appreciated her mother's attempt to educate her, but it left her just as bewildered afterward as she had been before.

> My mother is a nurse. She explained it in medical terms when I was about nine or ten, and I didn't even understand a thing she said. I mean, it was all over my head. Only a doctor, I think, could have understood it the way that ... she gave it a nice try! The way she explained it, it was only something you did when you wanted to have a baby ... it was like a shot. He—like in terms of a shot—would inject the sperm ... Really, until the first time Rex and I goofed up—that was the first time that I ever knew what it was really about.

Whether or not sex had been discussed in the home, the girls had been fully aware of their parents' attitude toward it. If parents considered sex "dirty" or "sinful" their daughters absorbed these attitudes. As Wanda knew so well, the effects of this kind of teaching were long lasting.

> My family was very ... these things were kept quiet ... "You don't do that. If you do that you are bad."
>
> See, here I have two kids, and I still have a very hard time thinking that sex isn't bad.

If parents had failed to provide information about sex, did the girls have a chance to get the basic facts in their schools? Good, comprehensive courses had usually been available only to juniors and seniors in high school. Some girls had received no instruction whatsoever in school, at any grade level. The majority remembered seeing a film in sixth grade or junior high.

I think if they would explain it more, and take more time with it, and let kids ask questions and stuff, instead of showing the film—and that's it—no discussion or nothing ...
What grade was that shown in?
Let's see ... the seventh grade, the eighth grade, and the ninth grade.
The same film?
Same film. The teachers make it like, "Sit down and watch the film, and then when it's over, you go back to your other work." That's it.

Ironically, the girls reported that the instruction which they had been given in the special classes provided for them *after they became pregnant* was of the highest quality—interesting, detailed and thorough—and it was really too bad they had had to be pregnant in order to receive it.

At the special class for pregnant girls they showed really good films, you know, on contraception and everything. At the junior high school they don't. I guess they figure you're too immature, or they just want to cover the basic things. And junior high school and high school is when a lot of girls start having sex. And they don't really know that much.
What grade were you in when you started having sex?
I was in the ... going into the seventh grade.

Their growing sophistication regarding relationships with men, and their increased understanding of sex and reproduction, made the girls realize how serious had been their lack of knowledge about birth control. Many stated emphatically that if they had only known more, they would have used contraceptives. Keeping control of their lives by this time seemed very important. The following comment was typical.

I would have gotten on the pill. If I knew all that I know now, *everything* would be different.

One girl remarked that she just couldn't figure out how she could ever have been so naive.

One of the reasons why I got pregnant to begin with was because, like a dumb female, I listened to what my boy friend said, because I was so much in love with him, you know, or cared about him and all that baloney, that he asked me not to take birth control pills! Next ... if I had it to do over again, I'd tell him to go fly his kite, *I'm not going to get pregnant!* If I can't take the pill, then — "*You* use something!" *That* — I think I would do that over!

All of the girls felt that they had grown up fast — because they had to. They had given up quite a bit, and other people had had to make sacrifices along with them. The knowledge and insight they now possessed had been acquired the hard way — by experience — and the cost had been high.

When they were asked if they thought the only way to learn was through experience, they replied emphatically that it was not. While admitting candidly that there are no doubt some people who learn only through experience, they maintained that for the great majority there is a much better way — *education,* and their ideas on this subject were fresh, thoughtful, and comprehensive.

First of all, there was unanimous agreement that everyone has the fundamental right to full and explicit information regarding sex and reproduction.

They felt, however, that no discussion of sex would be effective unless a great deal of consideration was paid to the importance of interpersonal relationships. This would have to include discussions by boys and girls together of subjects like exploitation, self respect, and the honest communication of feelings. It was this feature they had found lacking in almost all classes offered by schools.

I think it would be good to say the real things that happen — what a guy says to a girl, their emotion behind it, and stuff like that. They should not just teach the sex organs and how they work, that doesn't really ... that goes in one ear and out the other.

The girls stressed the importance of conveying to young people the idea that the act of intercourse was something very "special." Some of them had reached this conviction only after bitter experience, and it was one of these girls who made the following thoughtful statement.

I think I would tell young girls it's not all that fun ... sex, itself ... there's a lot more involved in it than just the physical act, and it can mess up your whole life. With all this sexual freedom and stuff, I think in a lot of cases that's the big thing—to be totally free, and to go with whomever you want.

But then you start losing your self respect, you start losing your identity, and you start wondering, "Well, who the heck am I?" You know, this really happened to me. I thought, "What am I? Am I just here for guys' pleasure?" And I really felt that's all I was here for, and I developed a nasty reputation. And I was not a nasty girl—I wasn't a loose dresser or whatever—I was a nice kid, you know, but I developed a really bad name.

It's miserable, it's really miserable for everybody in town to know you, and for your parents to find out about you from other people, you know ... they didn't believe it, but ... and then to have strange guys call you up for a date when they find out about you. It's miserable, it's really miserable.

And then when you go out with a guy that you really, really like, and you don't want—you know, you've *had* your experiences, you've put them behind you—you don't want to get involved with that, and the guy thinks, "Well, she's easy ..." It's really depressing to go out on a date with a guy you really like, and all you do all night is wrestle ... you know, in-the-back-seat type of thing ... And it's not fun, it's not all that fun. It may be exciting the first couple of times, or maybe the first time—I don't know—but it's awful darn hard!

They felt that boys needed to be as fully informed about pregnancy and childbirth as the girls, and that their education in this respect had been seriously neglected in the past.

They stressed how important it was that all young people receive instruction to prepare them for their future role as parents. They felt the schools should offer courses in child development and child rearing to all students—not just "the expectant mothers and the girls that already have kids."

They also pointed out that young people need to understand the legal and financial aspects of marriage, because those who had married young, expecting to enjoy their new freedom from parental restrictions, had learned the hard way that "along with that went the money, and the clothes, and—I don't know— you're just ... you're on your own." One of these girls said what most of them felt.

I think you need to know a lot. Marriage is like a closed book, really. You don't know until you get there.

Finally, just as they felt that everyone had a right to receive full information regarding sex and reproduction, they also believed that everyone had a right to receive the best possible instruction in methods of birth control. These young mothers knew from experience how poorly equipped they had been to deal with the kinds of social pressures that are prevalent today. It was Lynn, however, who made the most thoughtful comments on this subject.

I think that, first of all, if you feel like you're old enough to handle an emotional relationship, you need to think about some of the possibilities that you might encounter, and also make sure that the other person is ready to accept those same kinds of responsibilities. I think too many people ignore that before they get too deep into a one-sided relationship, before they find out that it's not what they thought it was. Also, I think that if you feel like you're ready for a physical relation- ship—if you're old enough for sex, you're old enough for birth control. If you feel like you're old enough to handle that kind of relationship, you're old enough to handle the responsibility.

Then she added a little advice for those who provide young people with information regarding birth control.

> I think if they would get off the approach, "Okay. We know you're doing it. We know you're doing it behind our backs. So we're making this information available to you," and say instead, "Okay. This may crop up in your life, so we'd like you to be prepared. We know that you're intelligent enough to handle it. If you can handle yourself in that kind of physical situation, you can handle yourself for being prepared," I think that would give some credit to kids.

Since all the girls agreed that young people need to have free access to all this essential information, if they are to be able to act responsibly and retain a certain measure of control over their own lives, then it became a question of who should provide the information. The usual sources of such information include parents, schools, girl friends, boy friends, and the street. Of these, the last three sources were definitely not recommended, since the girls who had relied on them had long since realized their mistake.

In view of the fact that only a few girls felt they had received adequate information from their parents, they did not think parents could be *counted on* to assume this responsibility. Although in some cases parents had broadened their viewpoint after seeing what one daughter had had to go through, this had not always happened. Jessica said her mother did not want her to discuss any questions about sex with her younger sister.

> She just don't want me to. She don't want her to know anything about it, because she thinks she's going to end up the same way. But she's going to end up the same way if she *don't* know anything about it.

The girls were aware of the embarrassment, lack of confidence, and anxiety which parents often feel when confronted by their children's need to talk about sex. But the sense of urgency they felt because of the pressures of today's society made them press for some way to meet the need. As they put it, *"Something somewhere has got to happen."*

Although very few had received more than token sex education in regular classes in the public schools, most of the girls spoke enthusiastically of the thorough instruction they had gotten in the special classes for pregnant girls. It was understandable, then, that they strongly recommended that the schools provide a comprehensive program of instruction for *all* students.

They tended to be impatient with parents' arguments against instruction in schools, and said their own parents had been willing to allow them to take such a course—or would have been willing, if such a course had been offered. They felt the young people were the losers in the arguments between parents and schools as to whose prerogative—whose right—it is to provide information about sex. One girl placed most of the blame for the impasse on parents.

> Parents are afraid of themselves. They don't want the schools to tell their kids—but they don't want to tell them either. But how are they supposed to find out but by experience?

Recognizing the obvious reluctance on the part of some school districts to become involved in sex education, however, another girl did not hesitate to call *their* bluff, so to speak. In discussing the common assumption that parents will probably not approve such instruction in schools, she spoke out plainly.

> Sure they will! The schools just don't try. I mean—I'm sure if everybody in this neighborhood came home and wanted to have a class, their parents would let them. The schools ... I think it's the schools that don't want to have it—not the parents. That's the way I figure it.

These young mothers, who knew what it was like to flounder along without adequate knowledge to guide them, and then be faced with a big responsibility too soon, refused to let differences of opinion cloud their thinking. They simply brushed aside all arguments against sex instruction in schools, with pithy comments such as this: "It's going to teach them a lot more than American History!" In fact, a great many felt schools should be required by law to provide such courses, and parental consent should not be necessary.

> I don't think there should be any parental consent. You don't need to have parental consent to have a child take a biology course, and to me sex education is vital. You *have* to be informed about this!
> What happens to the child at school is a learning process. That's what sex education is—it's a learning process.

Meanwhile, they were not sitting around waiting for society to allocate responsibility for sex education, but were rather taking whatever action they could themselves. Many had already talked with younger sisters, brothers, cousins, and friends, and some had spoken before classes at school, drawing freely on their own experiences to drive home their points. They did not mince words. Their message was clear and unmistakable.

> Wait. Wait until you've got your own pad and old man, groceries in the cupboard, got all your running done, and settle your ass down, and *then*—I don't care if you have a thousand kids!

CHAPTER FOURTEEN

Unfinished Business

Many readers have probably been thinking, as they listened to the young mothers telling their stories, "All these problems could have been avoided if they had only acted responsibly."

It is very easy, particularly for adults, to make such a remark and feel that the subject is closed. But it is *not* closed. Girls at ever younger ages will continue to bear children unless it is generally accepted that the responsibility for adolescent pregnancy is actually a *comprehensive responsibility* in which adults as well as teen-agers share.

Typically, adolescents are carefree, happy-go-lucky people, not noted for a highly developed sense of responsibility. Adults usually dismiss most teen-age highjinks with an indulgent shrug of the shoulders, as if to say, "Never mind. They'll grow up!" But when young people get mixed up in problems associated with sex, it's quite a different story. Why? Because adults have learned that sex *requires* responsibility. What they may not realize is that a great many boys and girls have been allowed to reach adolescence without ever having learned what responsibility really is.

Parents have an obligation to teach their children responsibility at an early age, so that by adolescence the *habit of responsibility* is well established and can be applied to attitudes toward sex. Parents also have a duty to make sure that their children are fully informed about the nature of sex *before* they have actually begun to engage in it. At the same time parents should realize that their own attitudes toward sex, and toward each other, will have a more profound effect upon their children than anything they say.

Schools, in turn, have an obligation to provide courses in the fundamentals of human sexuality designed to meet the needs of all students. To be effective, these courses should deal with the subject in a perfectly frank and natural manner, and no student should finish the instruction with his questions still unanswered. Such courses will always meet with some opposition, but schools should stand firm in defense of every student's *right to know.*

Two groups of professionals are especially qualified to help and advise young people in matters relating to sex—physicians and clergymen; but in actuality, many a family doctor, and many a minister, priest, or rabbi, has simply avoided dealing in a straightforward manner with problems of teen-age sex. As a result, young people have been seeking out free clinics and counseling centers in preference to consulting with their own doctors and clergymen. Since these services are not universally available, both the medical establishment and the churches need to take stock and consider how to win the confidence of teen-agers, and how to help them deal with problems related to sex.

The general public, too, has certain obligations. When confronted by reports that teen-age pregnancies are not only increasing in number but also involving ever younger girls, people should try to find out *why* this is happening, especially in their own communities, instead of giving way to feelings of exasperation and condemnation. If they are to be of any help to young people, they need to become familiar with the problems that young people face; and before jumping to any conclusions, they need to obtain factual information and compare it with the arguments of groups seeking to sway public opinion in one direction or another.

Those who represent the public in local, state, and national government also need to become familiar with both the problems and the facts, so that they can protect and defend the rights of young people—including their right to know, and their right to make choices. They, too, will have to distinguish between statements of fact and cries of hysteria, always keeping in mind the principle that individual responsibility can be *taught* but not *legislated.*

Finally, young people—both boys and girls—will have to get their facts straight, and realize that experimenting with sex is not on the same level as experimenting with drinking, or fast driving, or smoking pot, or any other "adventure" so attractive to teen-agers. Many of these experiences carry high risks—for the teen-ager or somebody else—of injury, or even death. But sex as an "adventure" is in a class all by itself, for it alone involves a risk that admits no comparison—the risk of accidental *life*.